How do I see a stereogram?

Would you like to see the reliefs hidden in these stereograms (3D relief images)?
Don't panic, here is a step-by-step guide to help you discover them.

You will have to be patient because when you are not used to deciphering this kind of image it is not always easy. You must forget your habit of staring at the same point with your eyes. The goal to see the relief of the hidden image is to have a parallel vision. (By staring at a point far behind the image).

The method to help you there:

First of all, almost stick your nose on the book and let your gaze "float" in the void as when you are tired and don't stare at a particular point or watch TV thinking about something else. Your vision should normally split slightly. Then bring the book close to your nose (about one hand distance) and then slowly and gradually move it away from your face so that the relief is revealed to your eyes.

With practice you will no longer need to stick to the book, you will know how far away you need to position yourself to discover the 3D images.

Have a little more patience! Soon, the stereogram reliefs will no longer hold any secrets for you.

This book is the second of its kind that I edit and I hope you will like it. Others will soon come out, be it stereograms or other mind games.

BE CAREFUL, ALL THE IMAGES TO DISCOVER INSIDE ARE LANDSCAPE, SO YOU HAVE TO TURN THE BOOK WITH THE FOLD ON TOP.

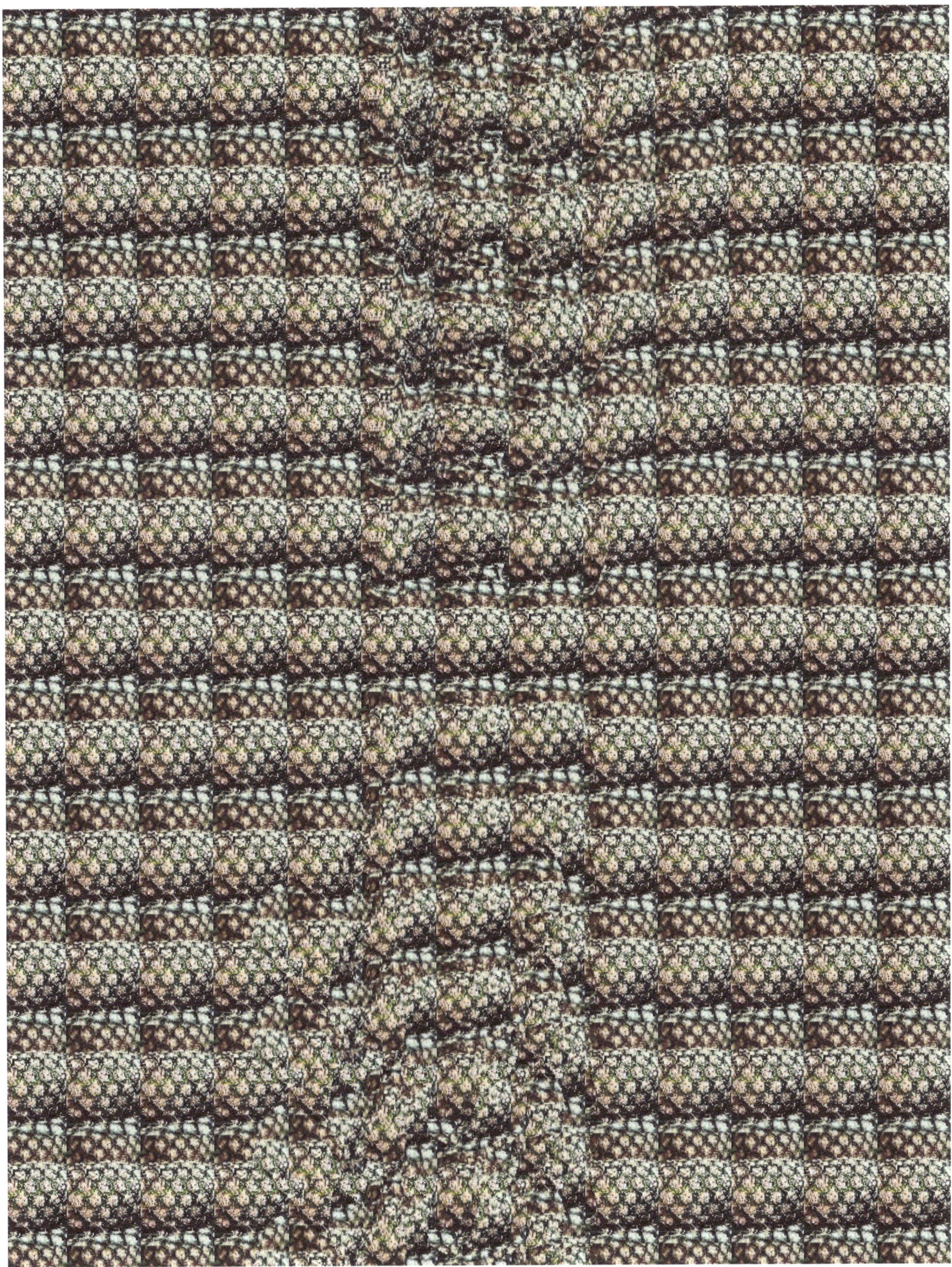

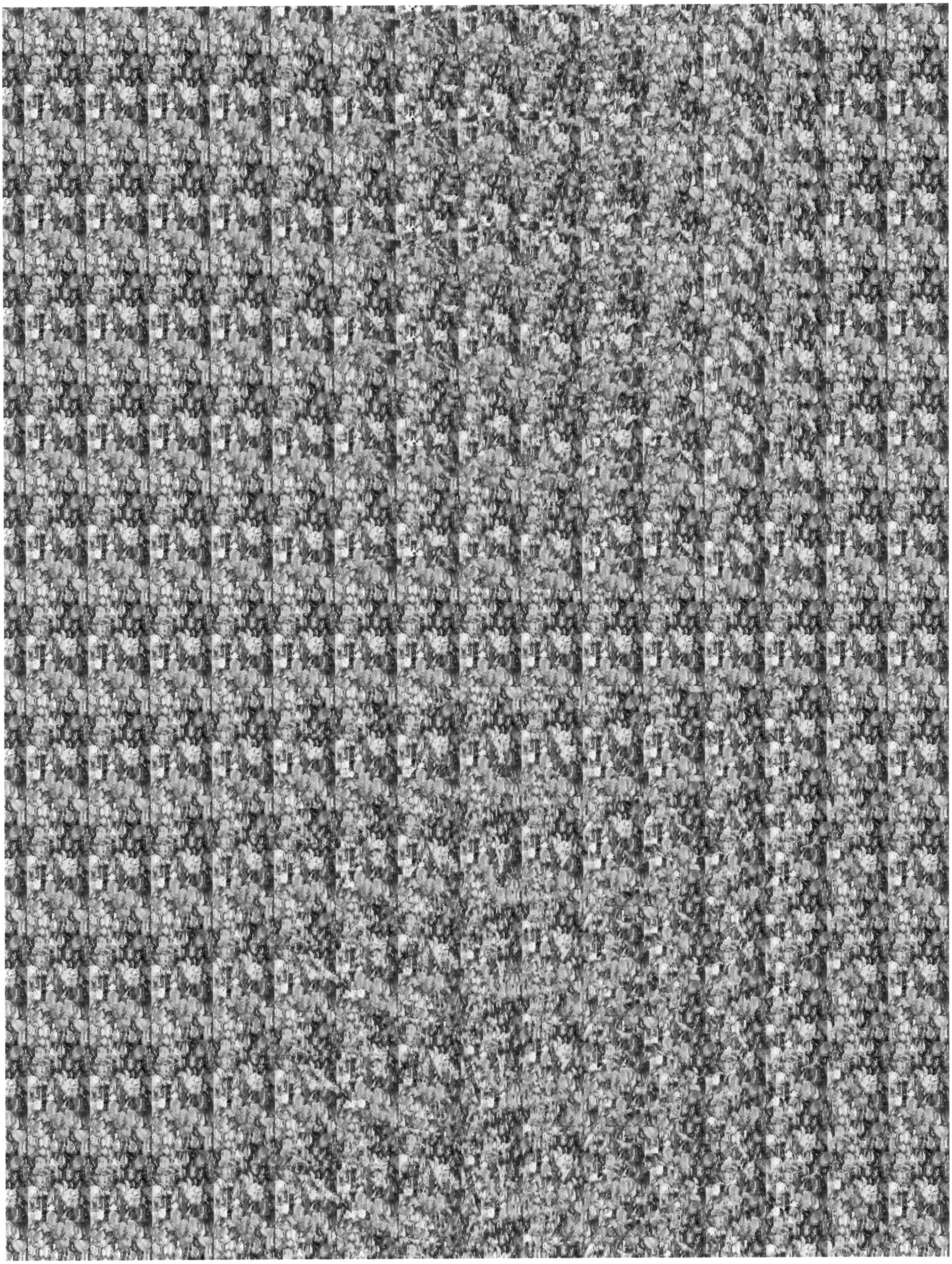

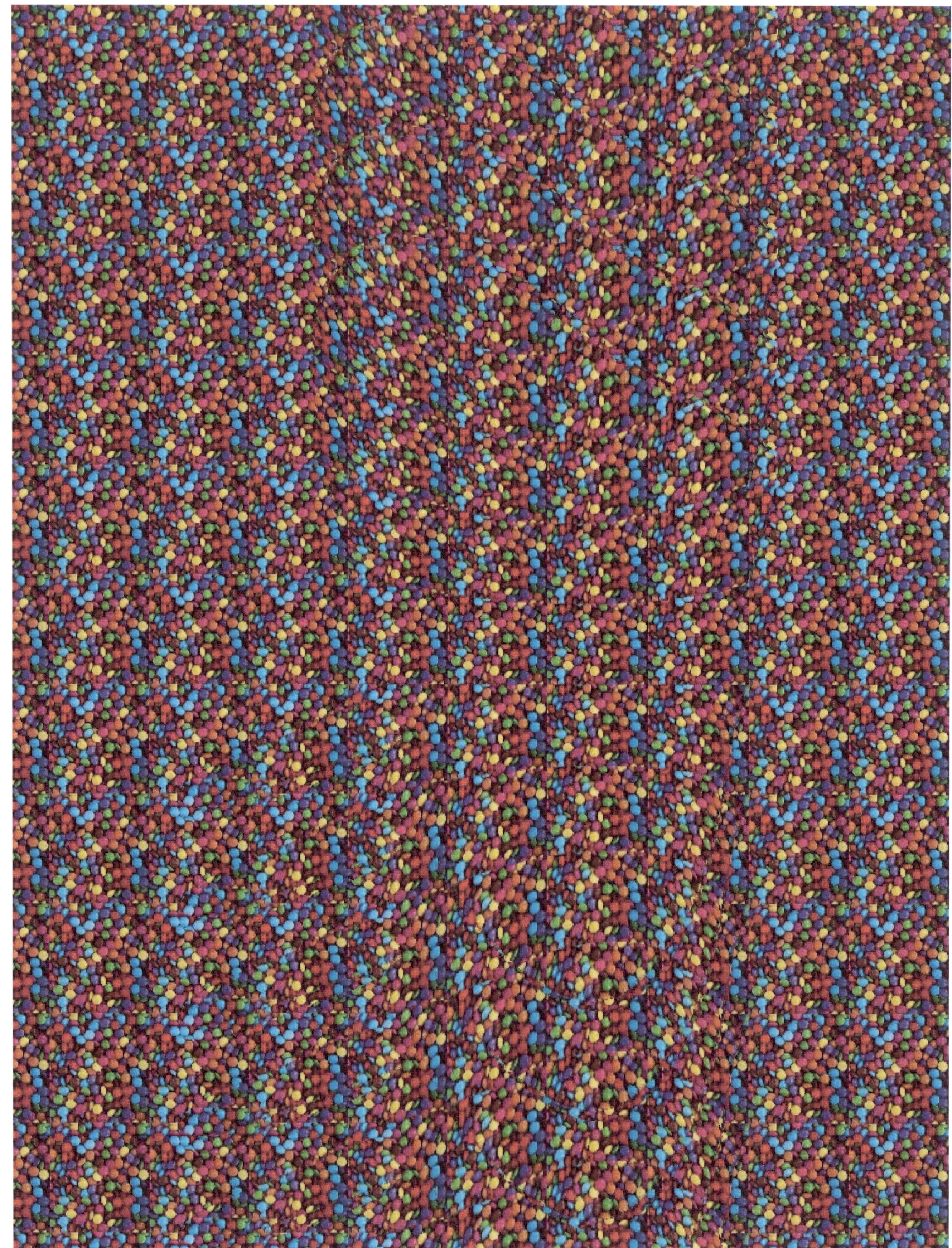

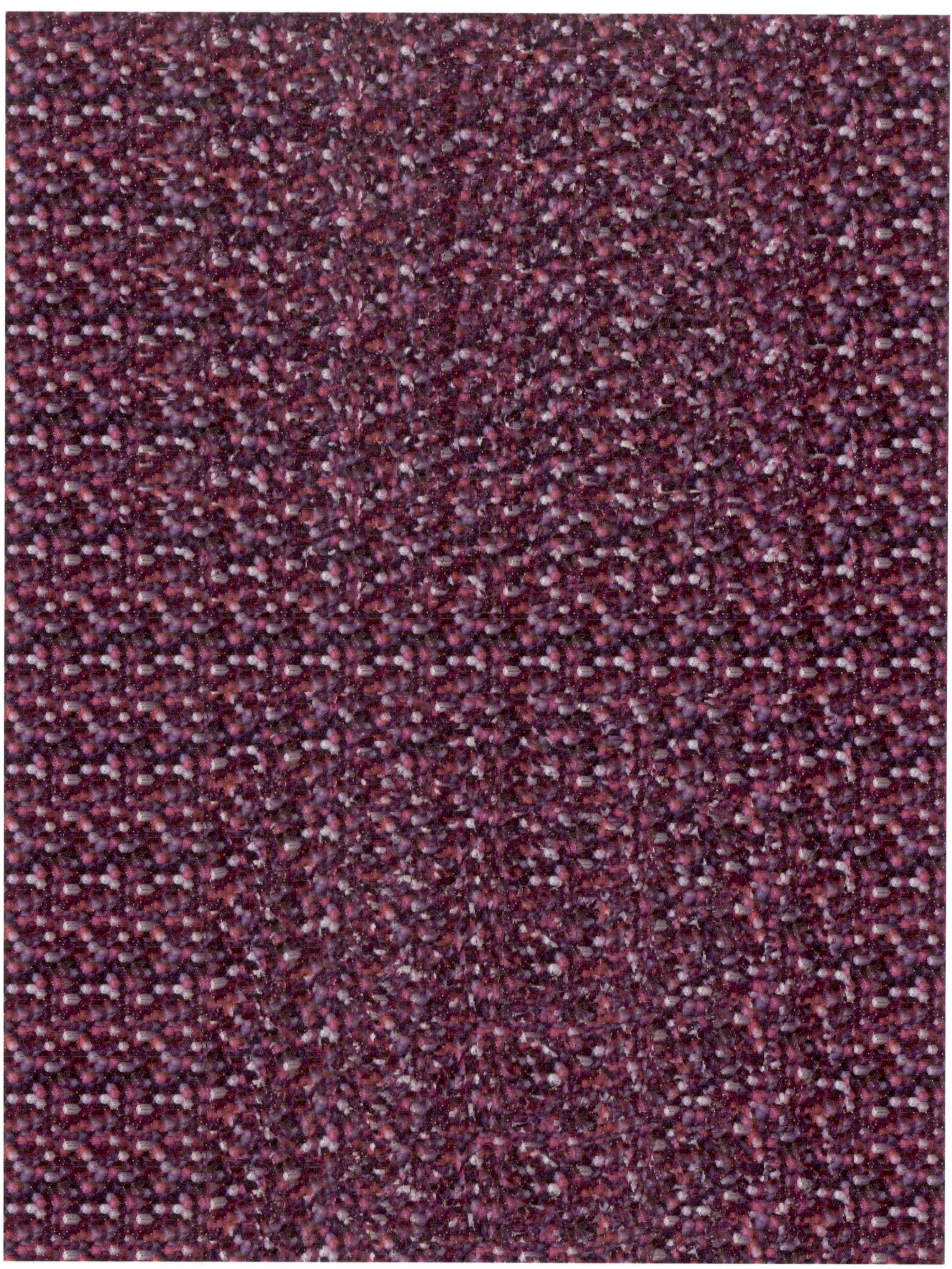

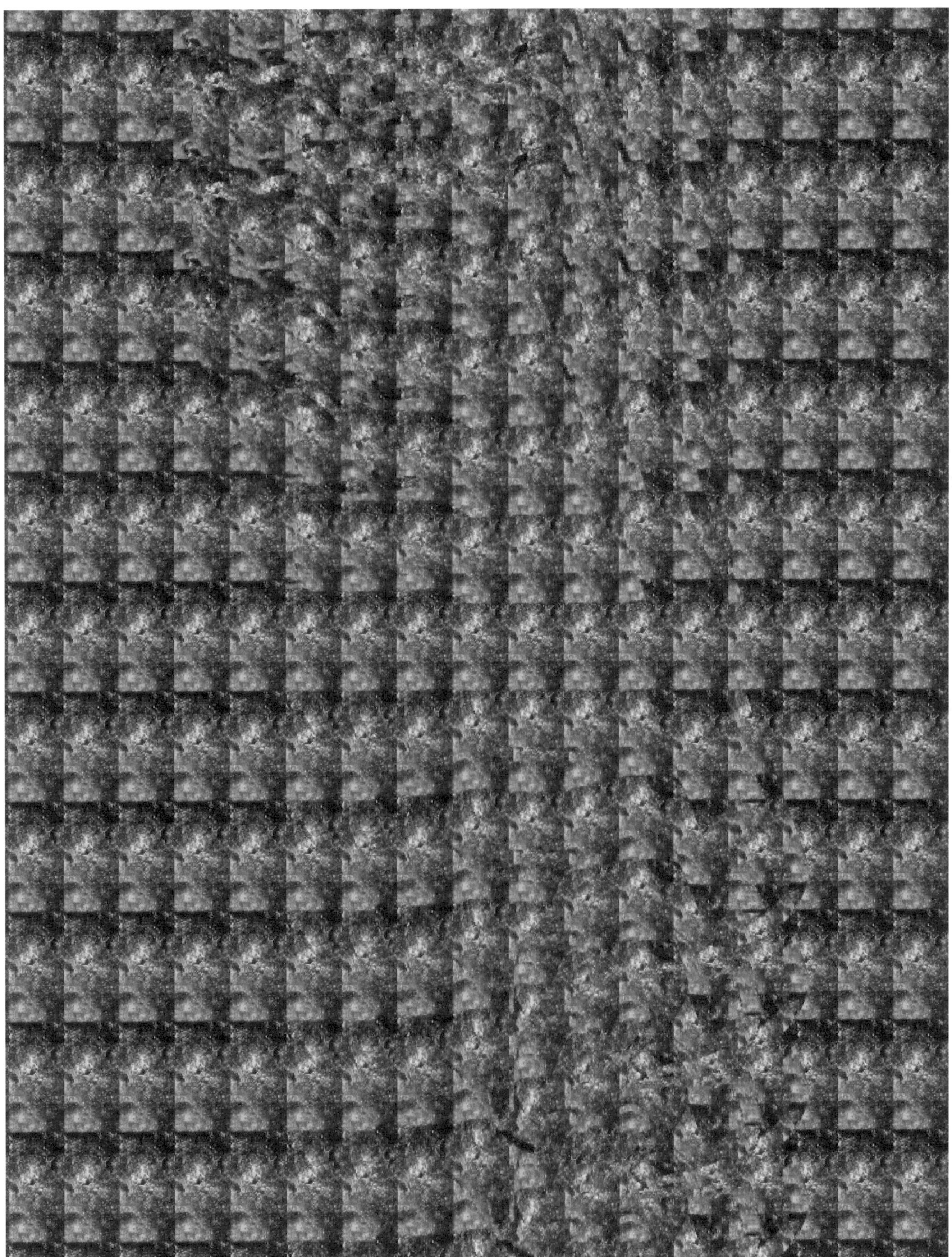

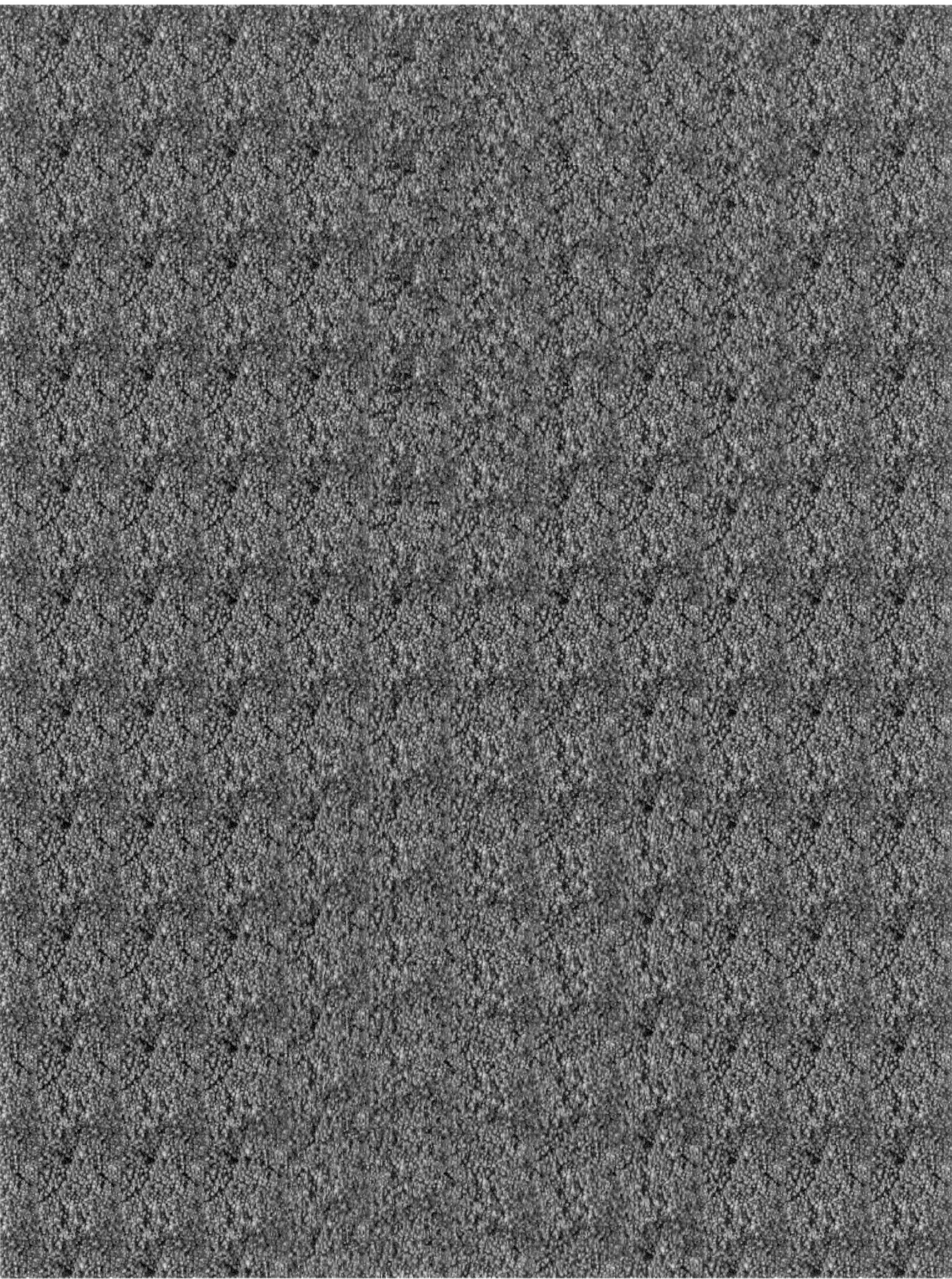

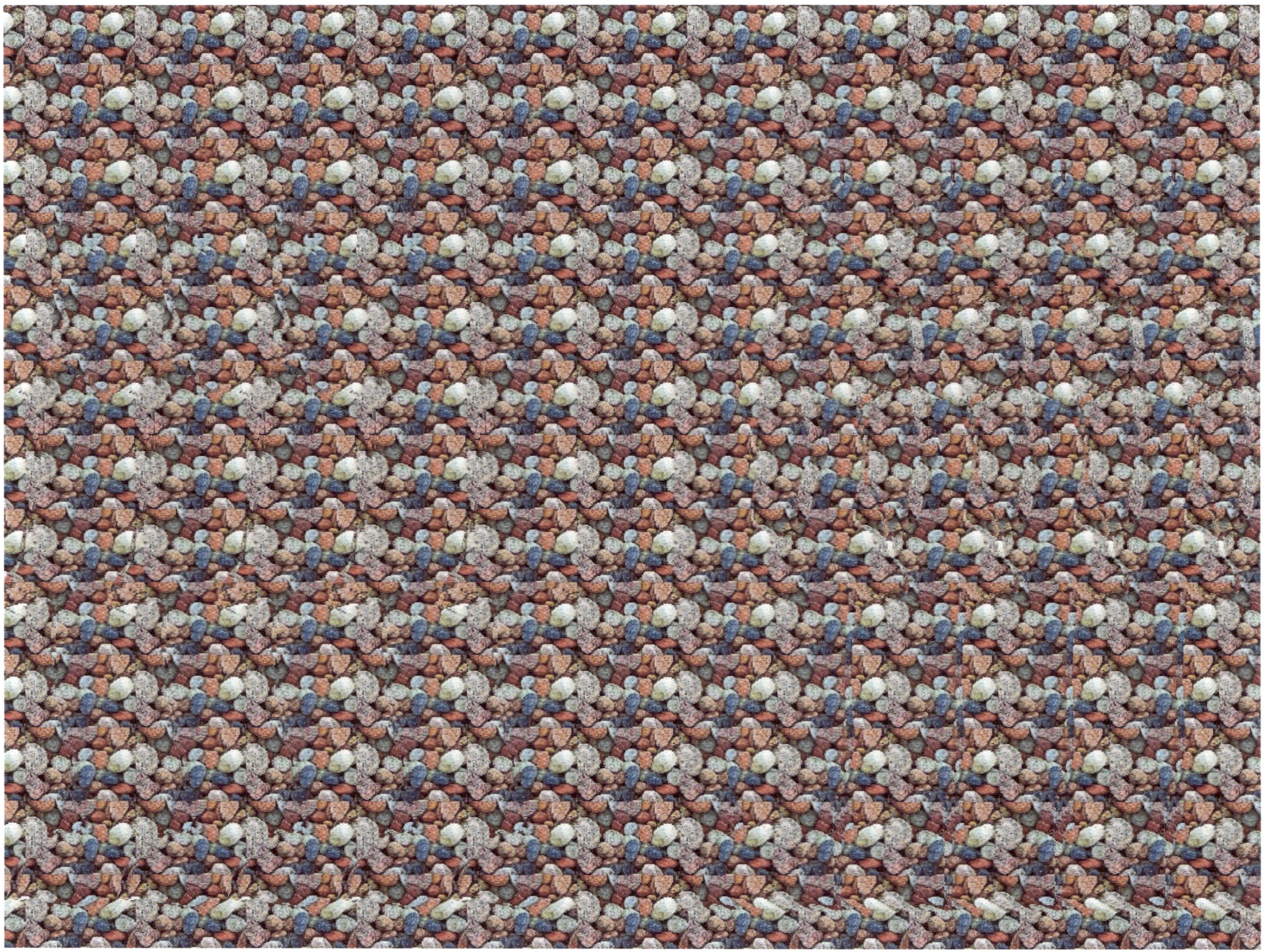

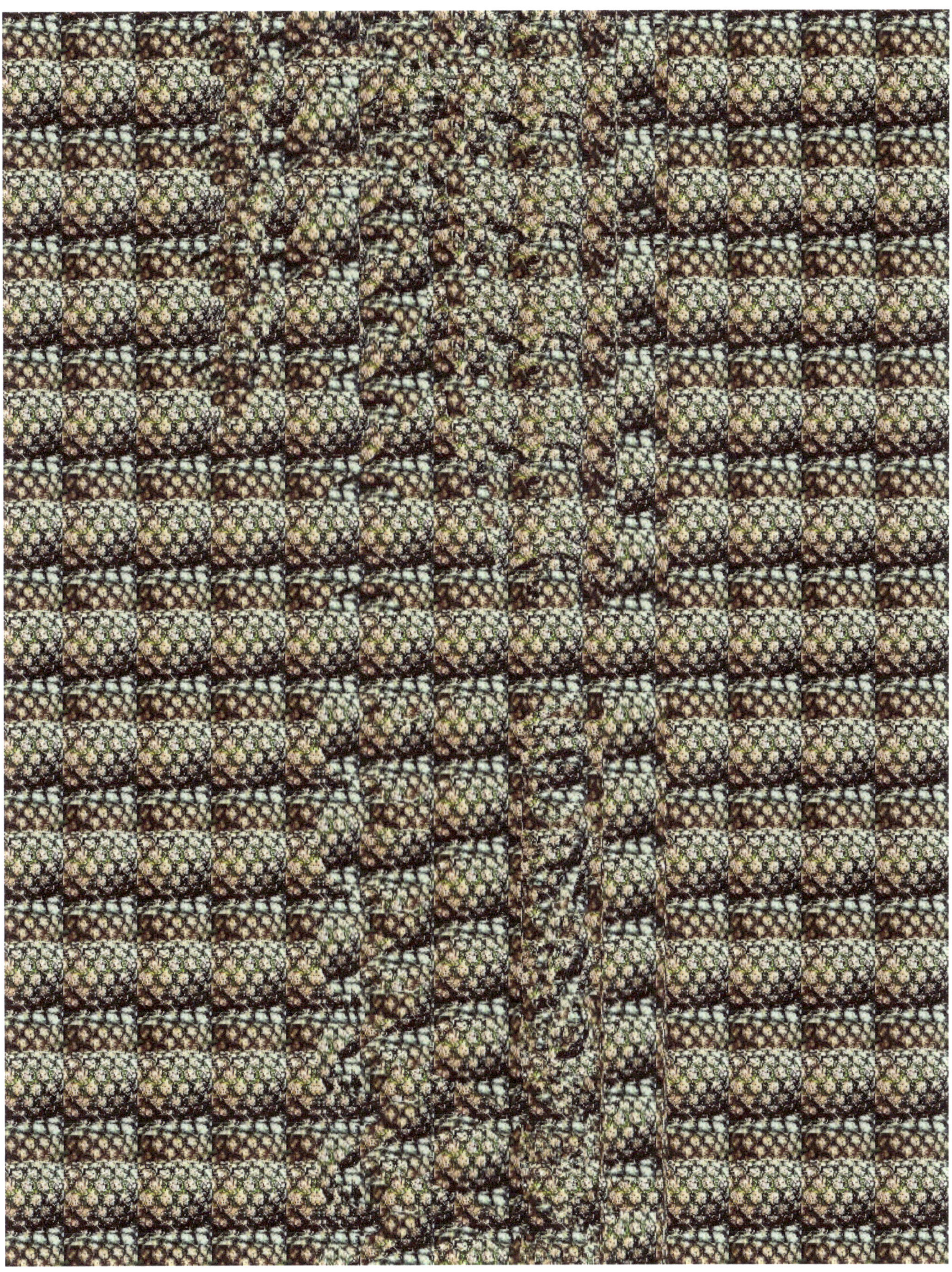

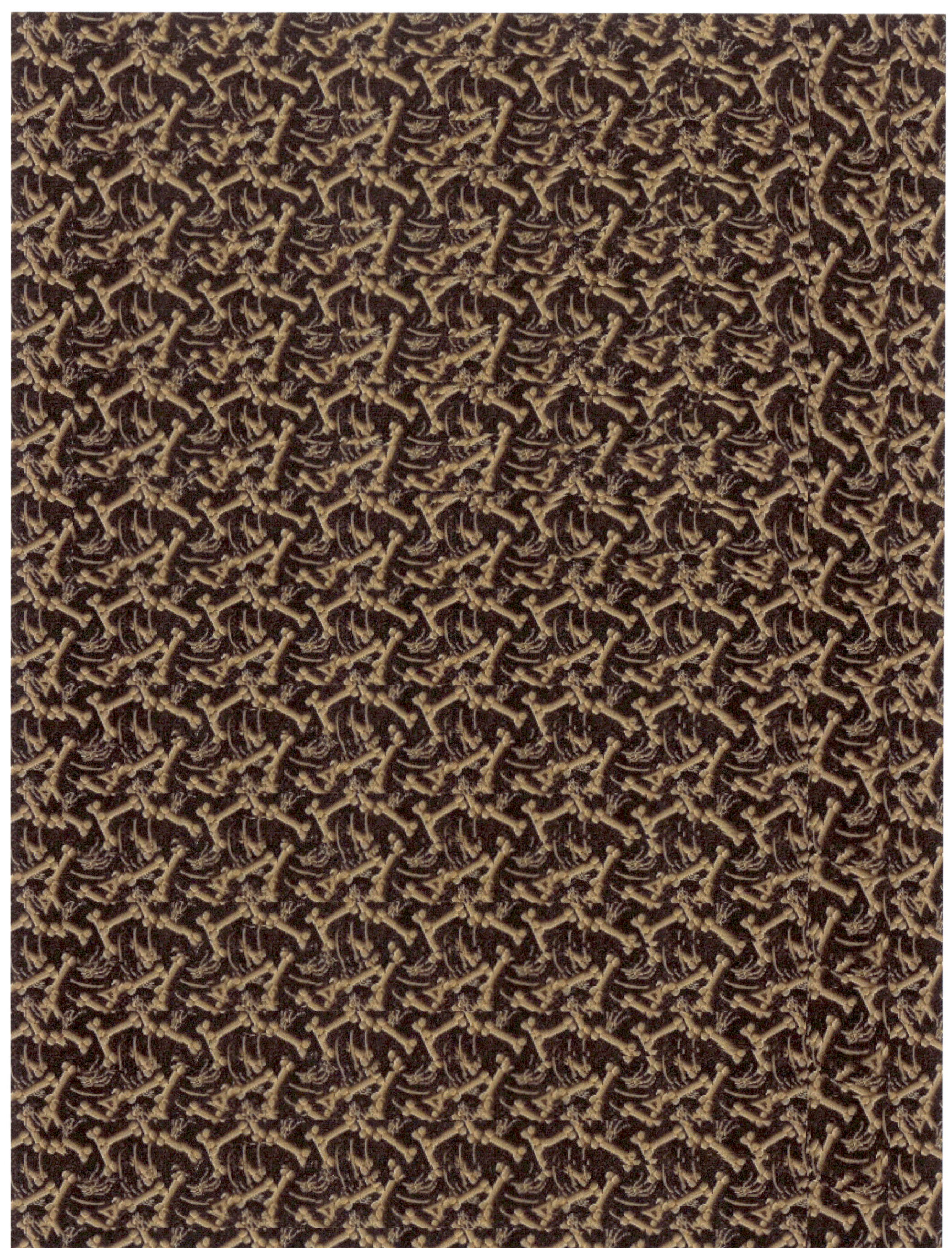

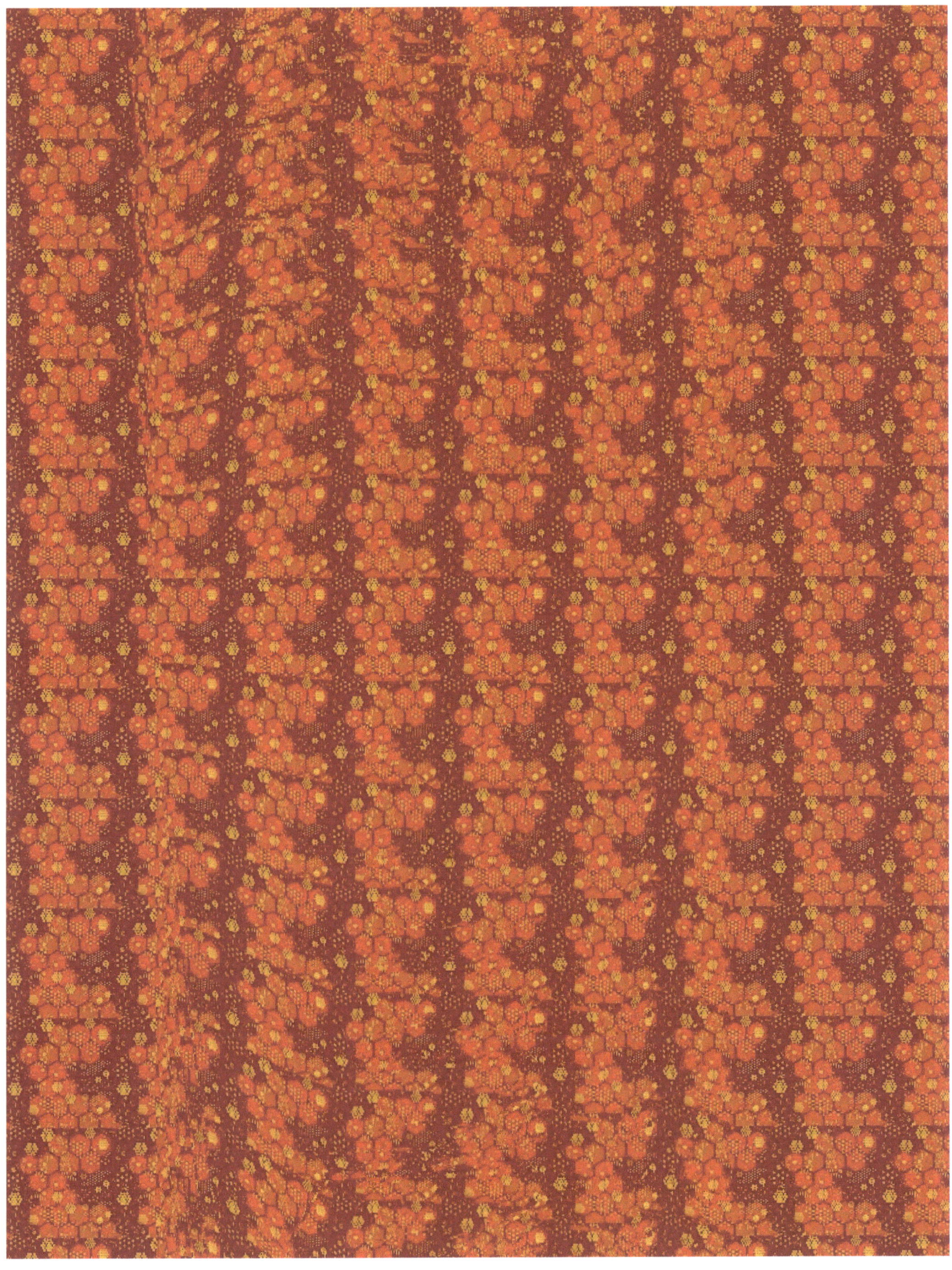

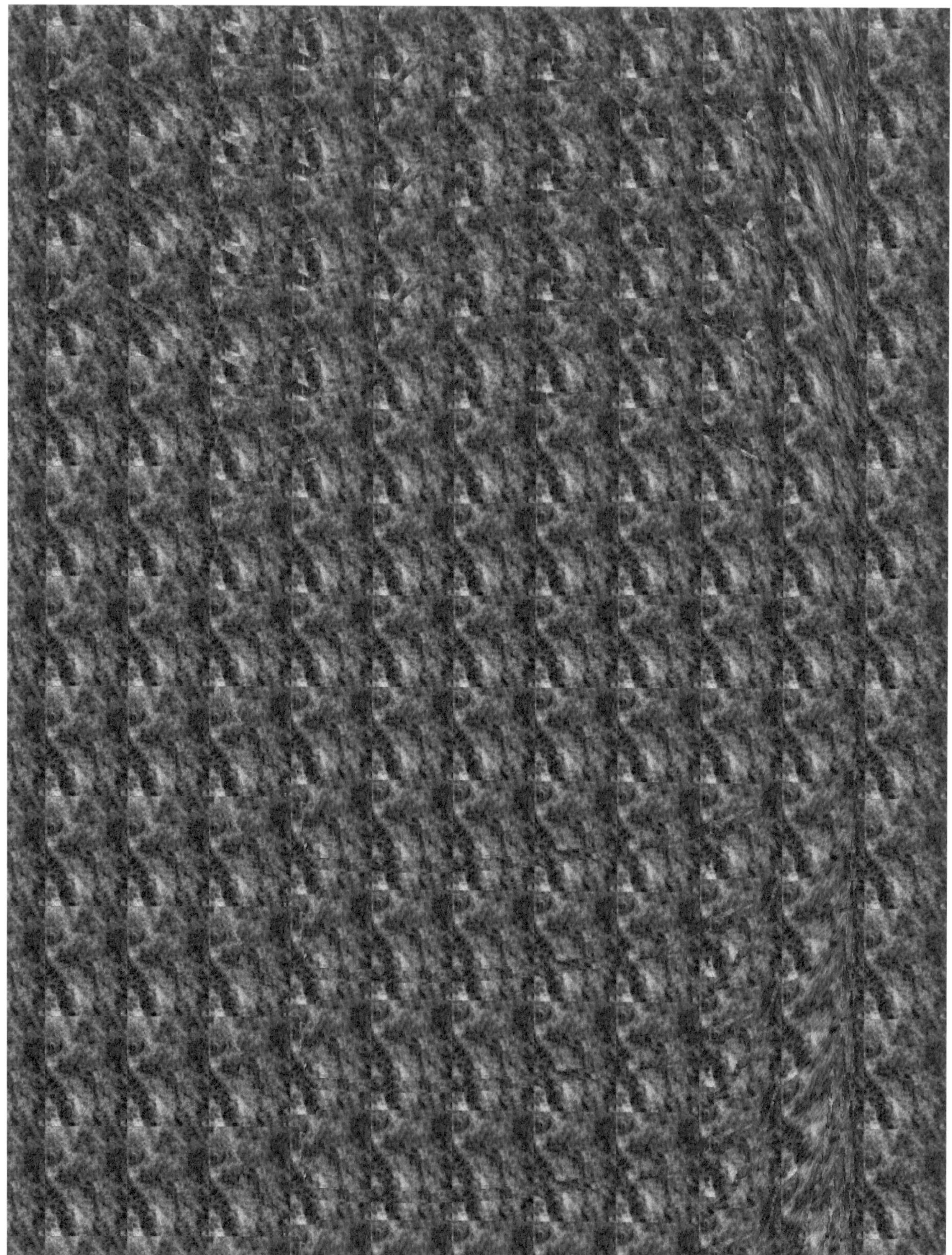

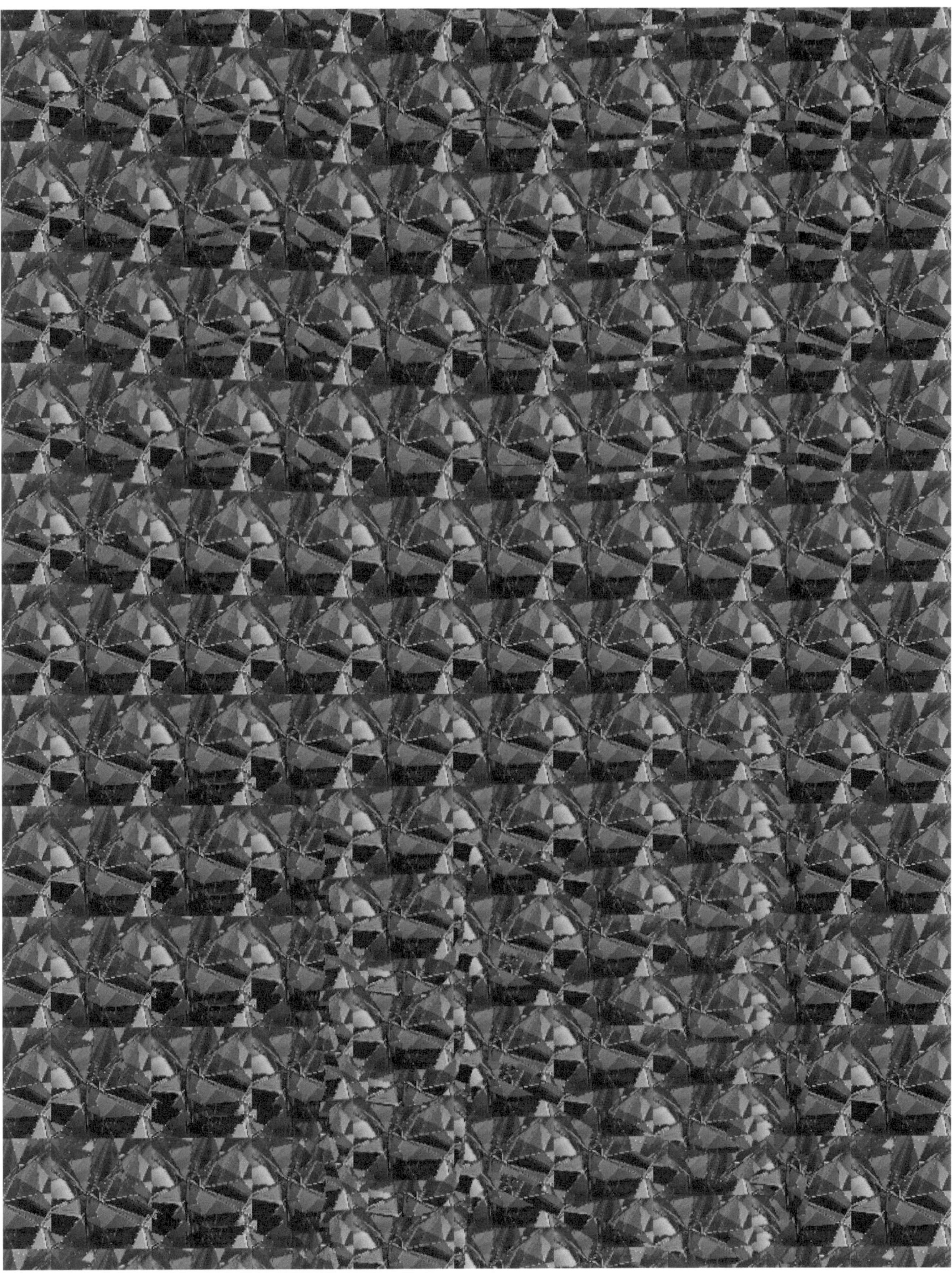

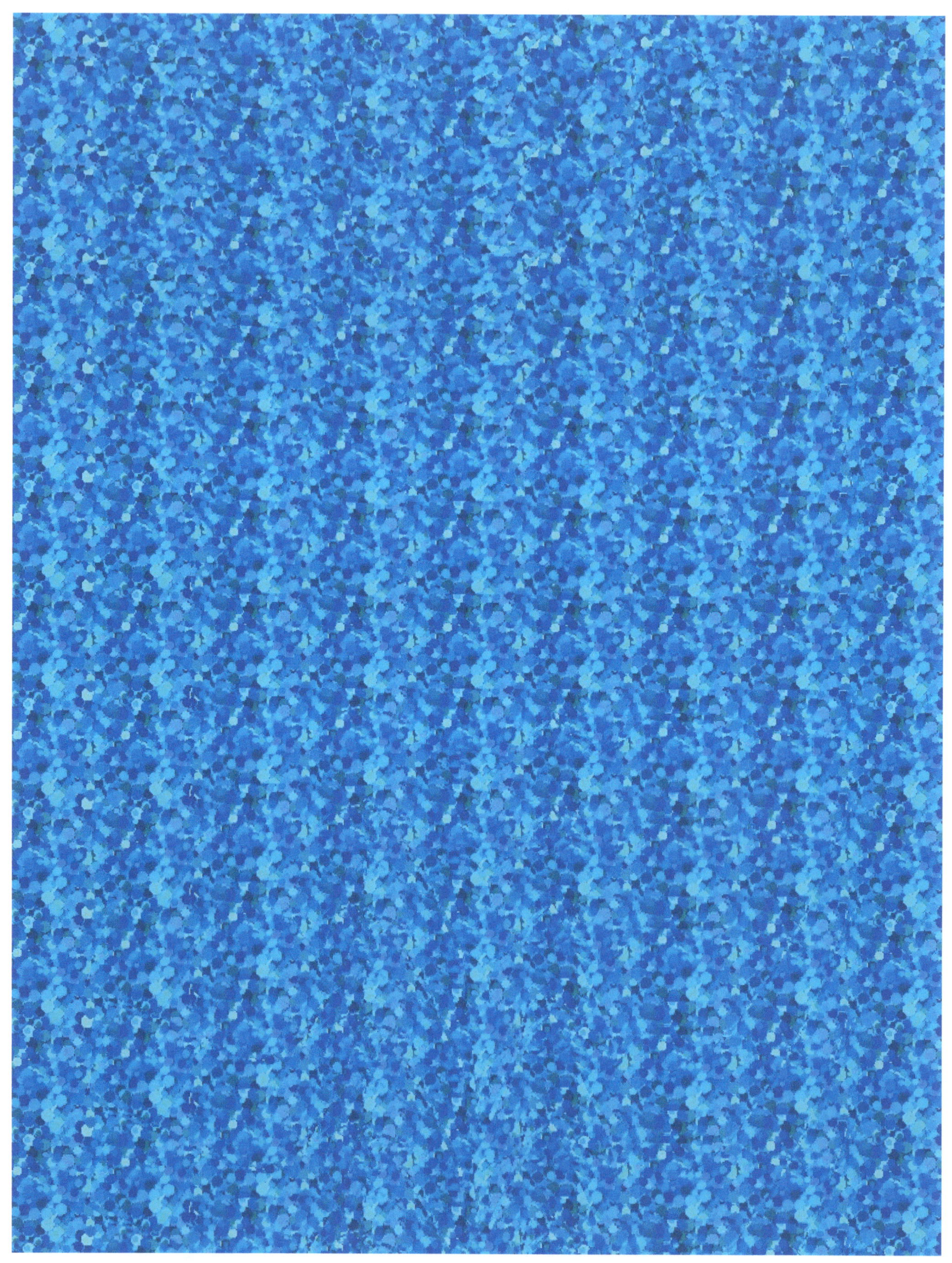

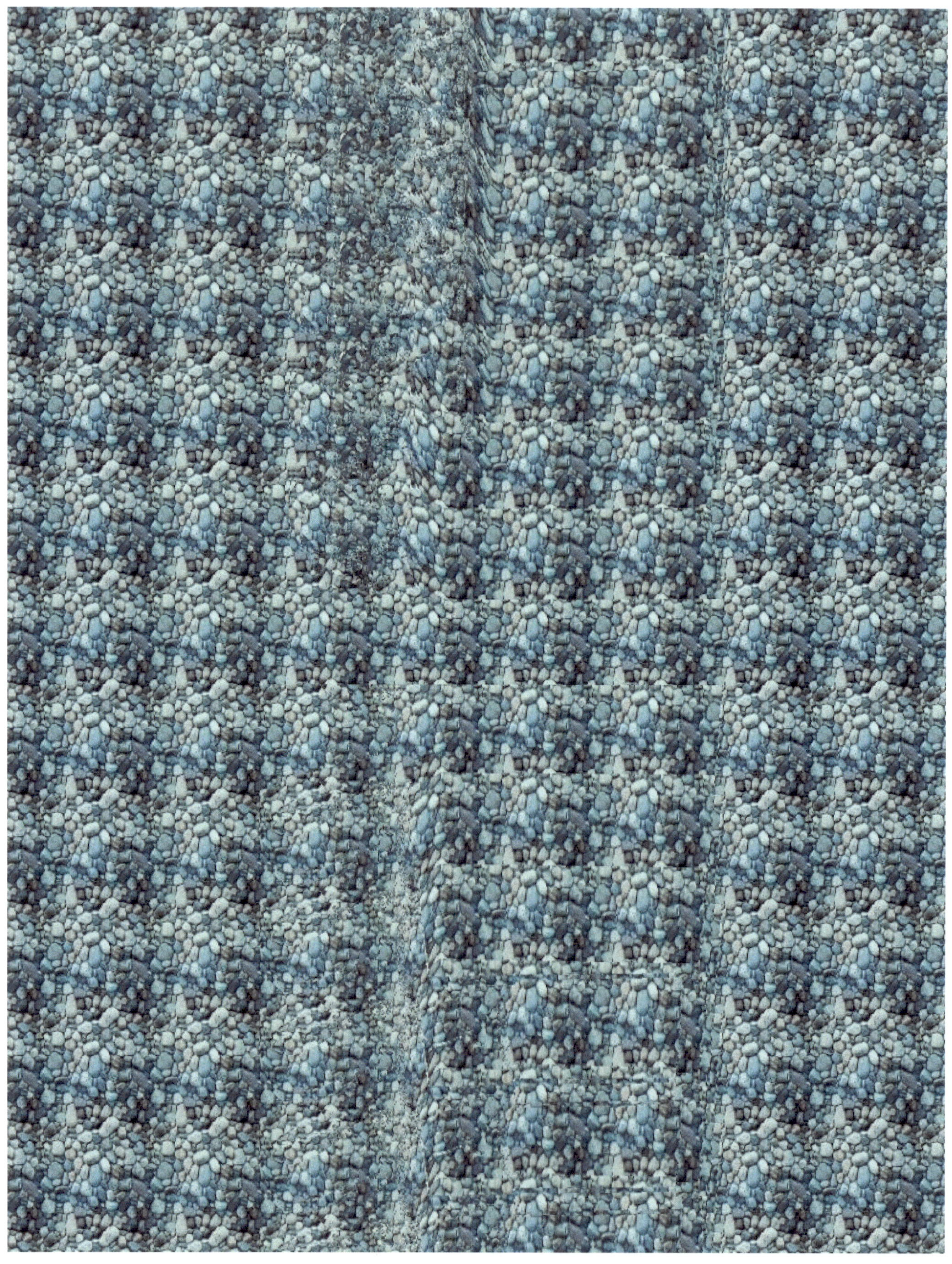

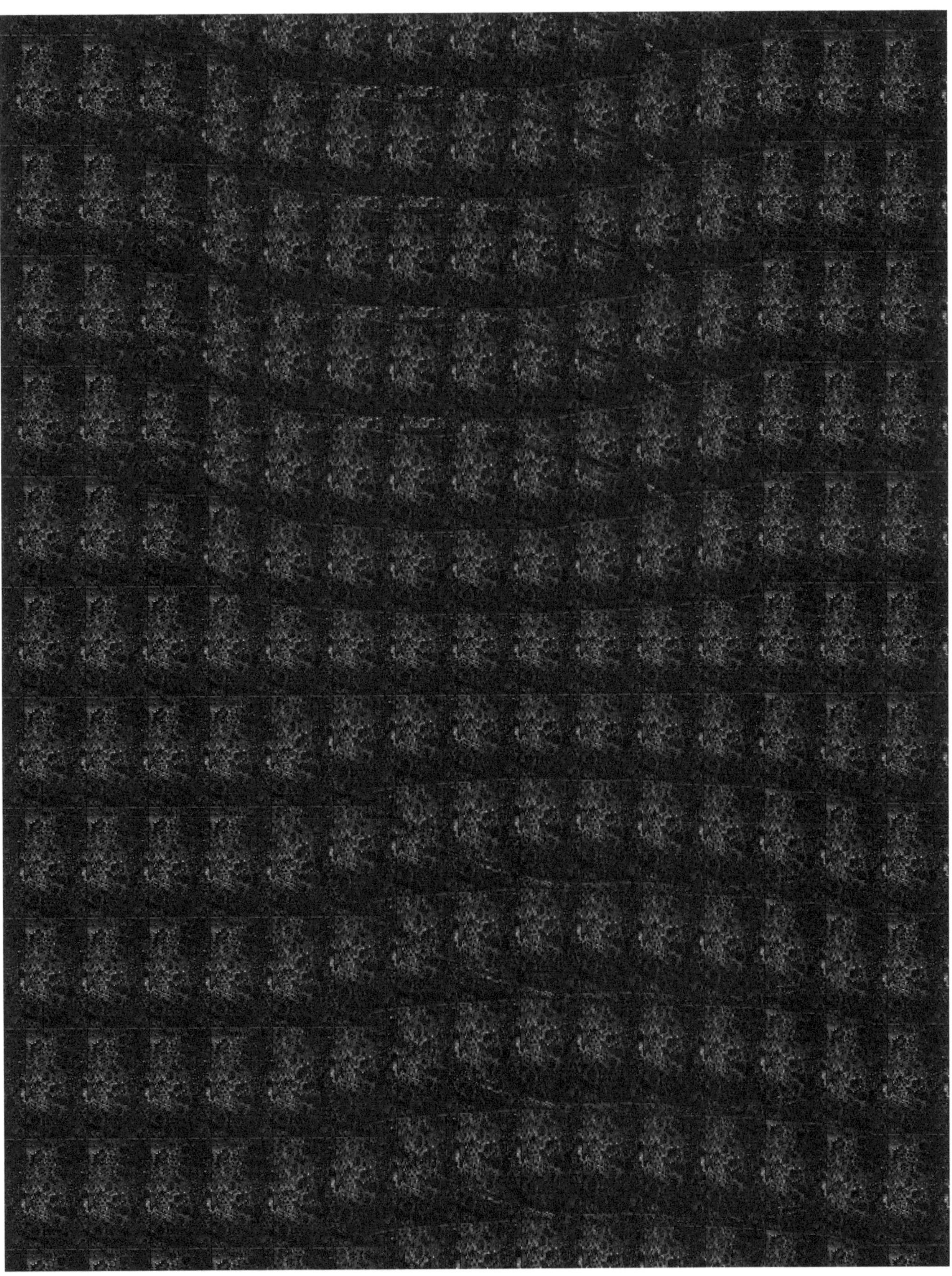

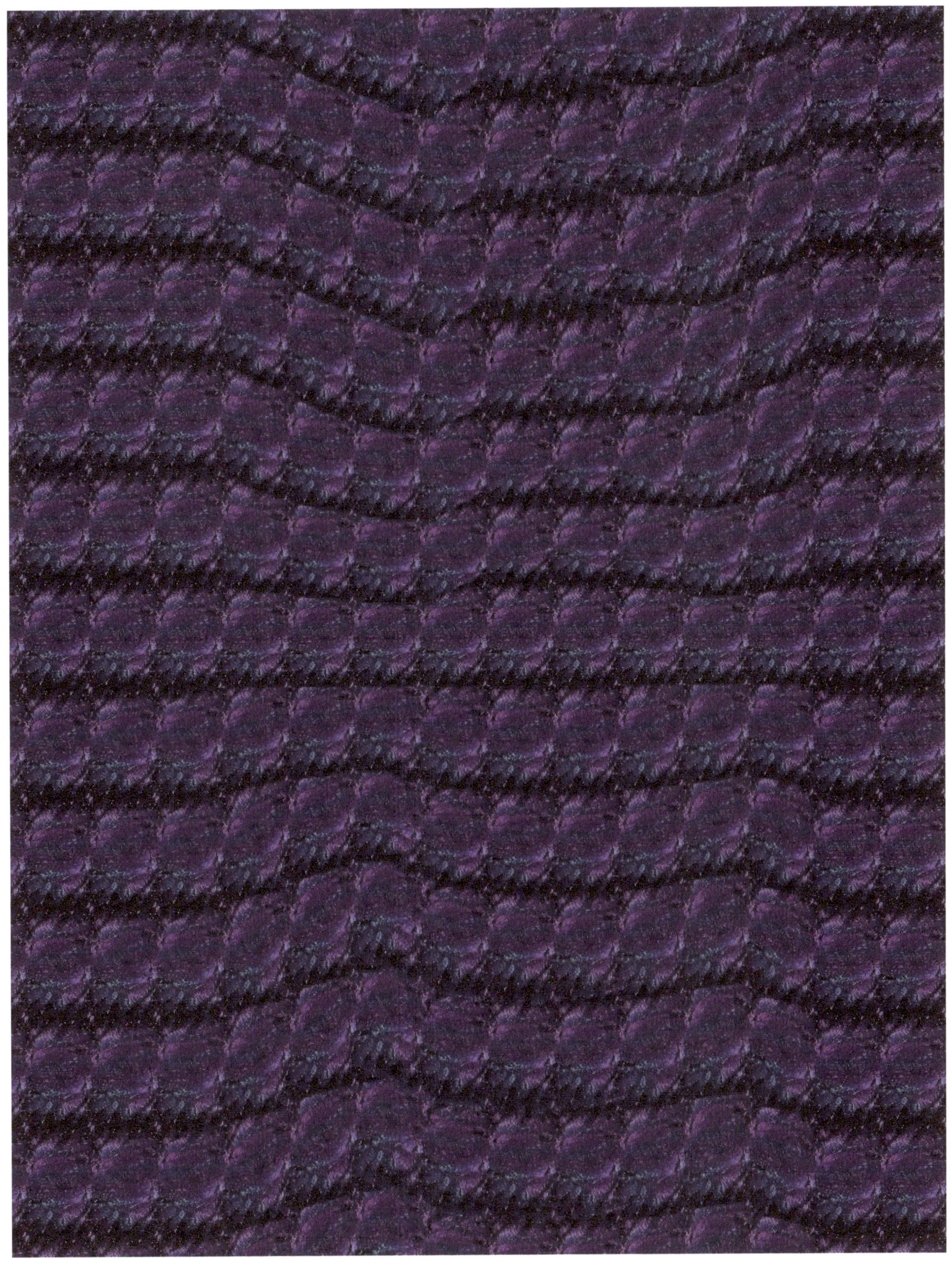

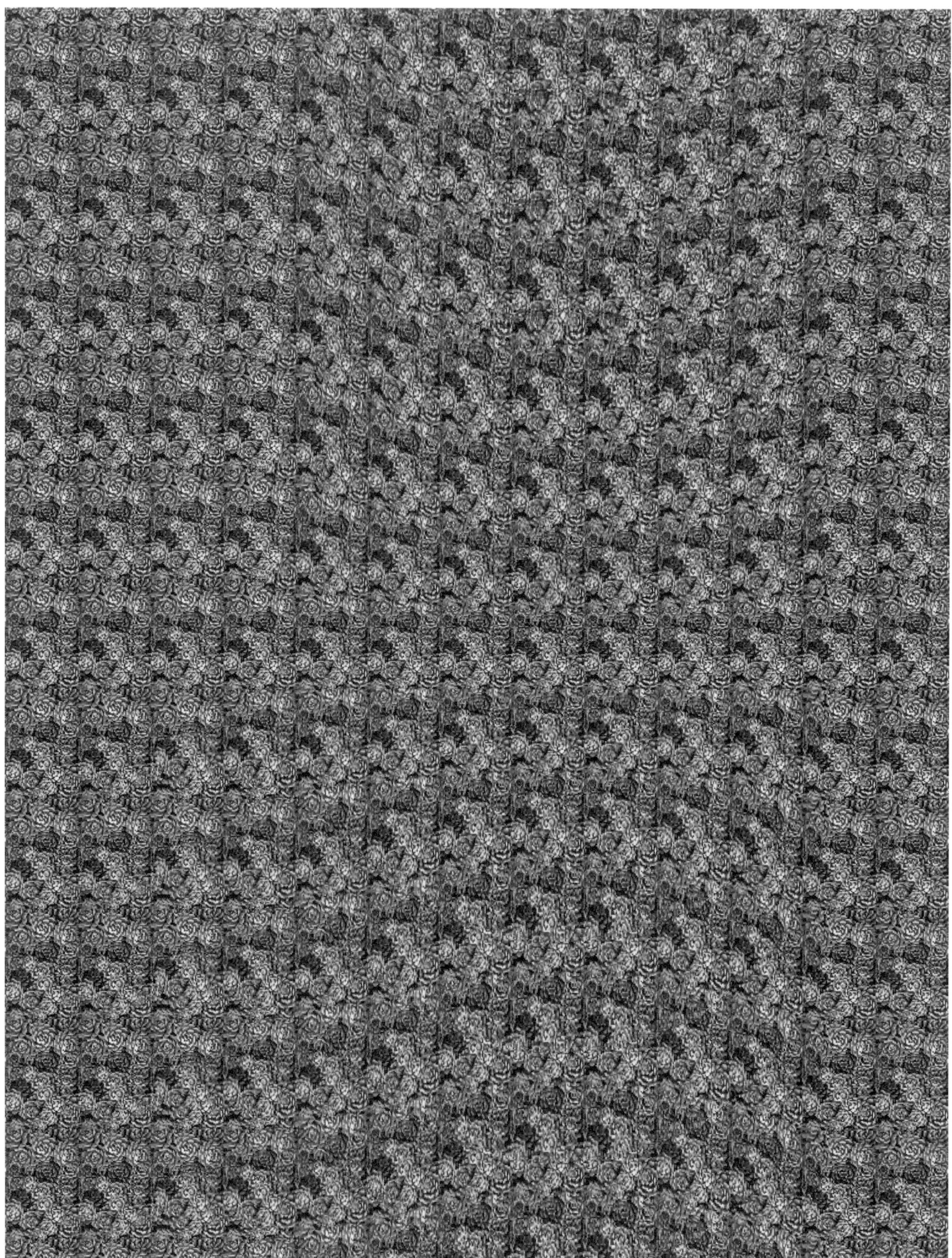

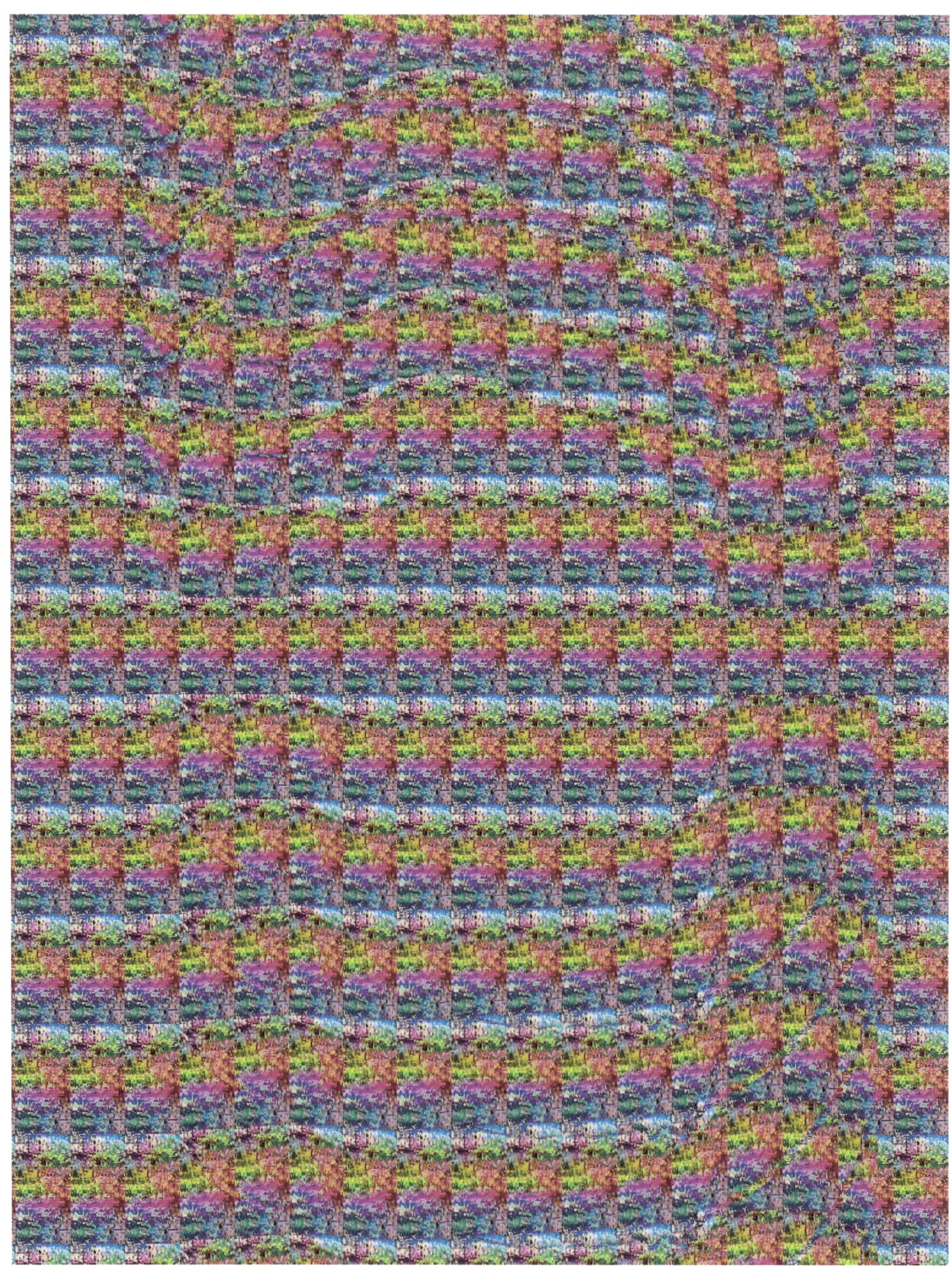

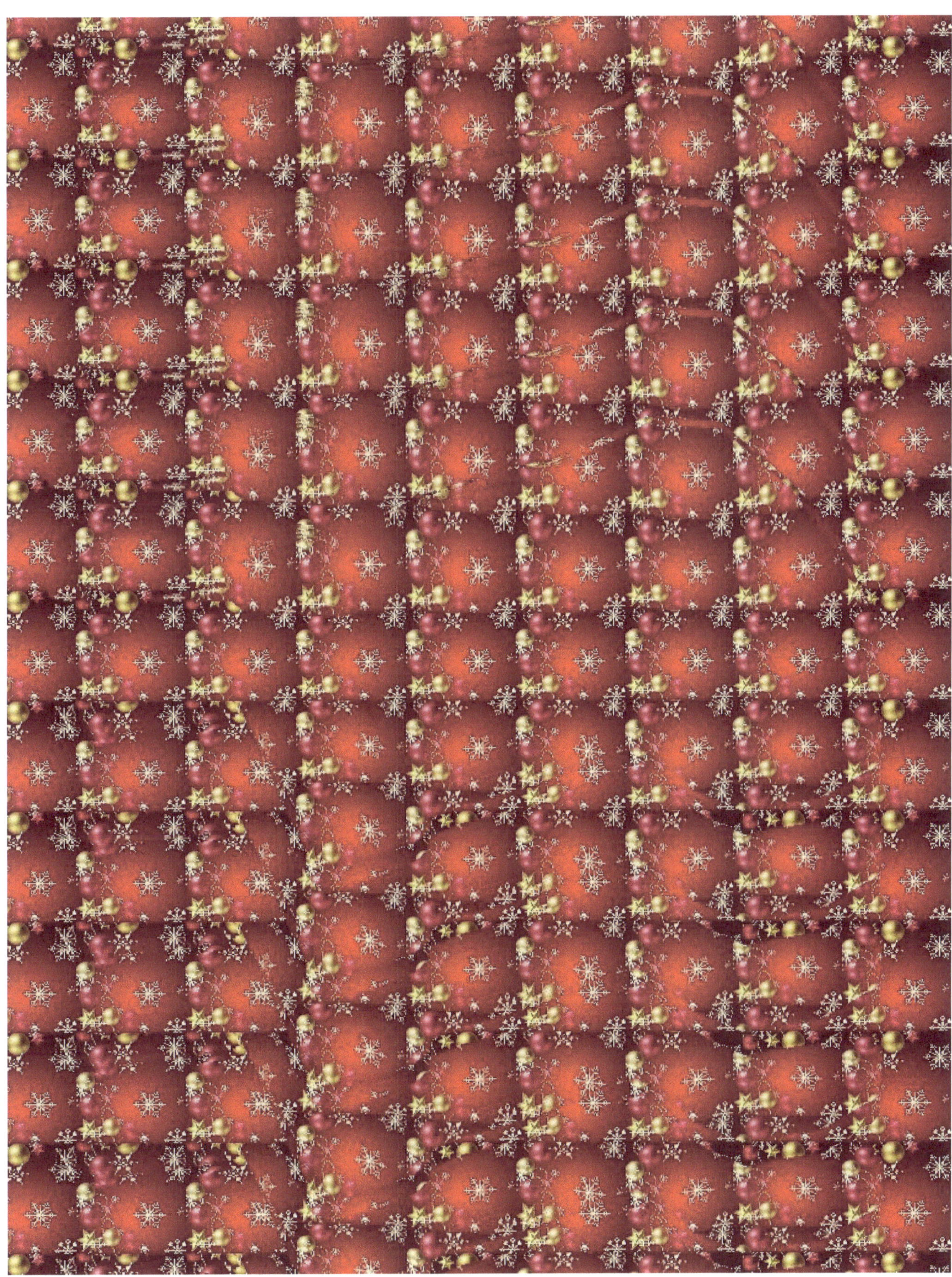

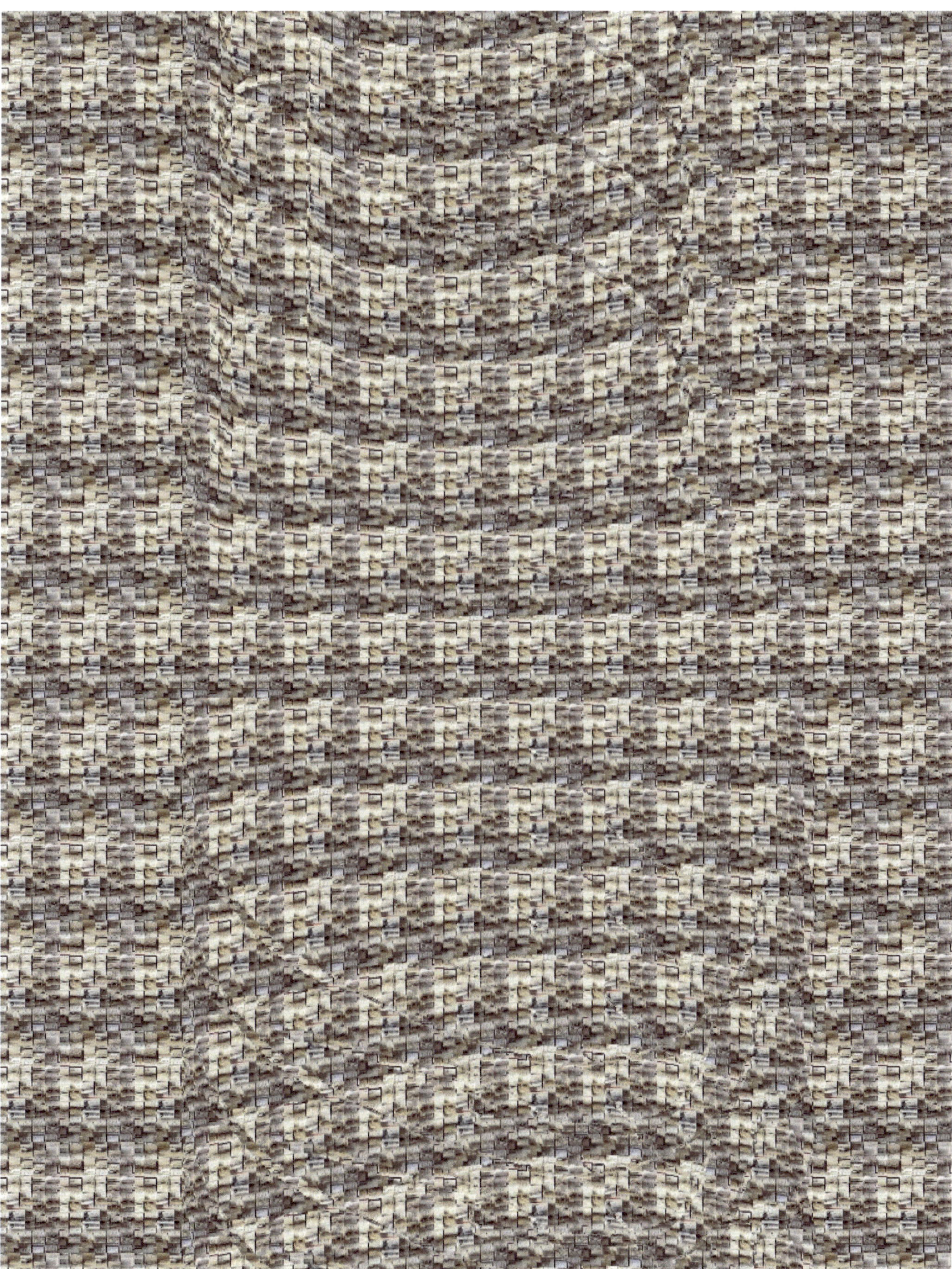

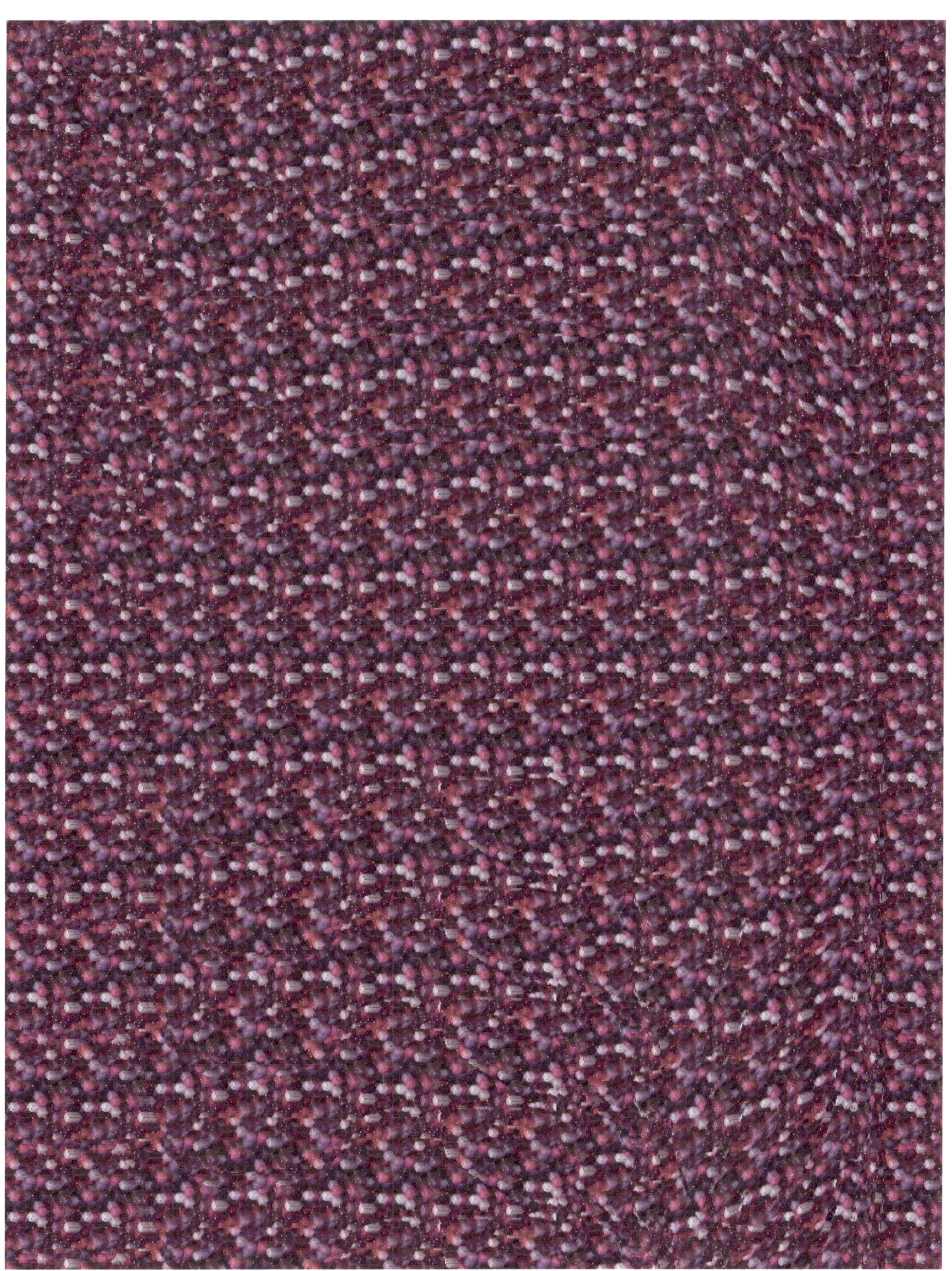

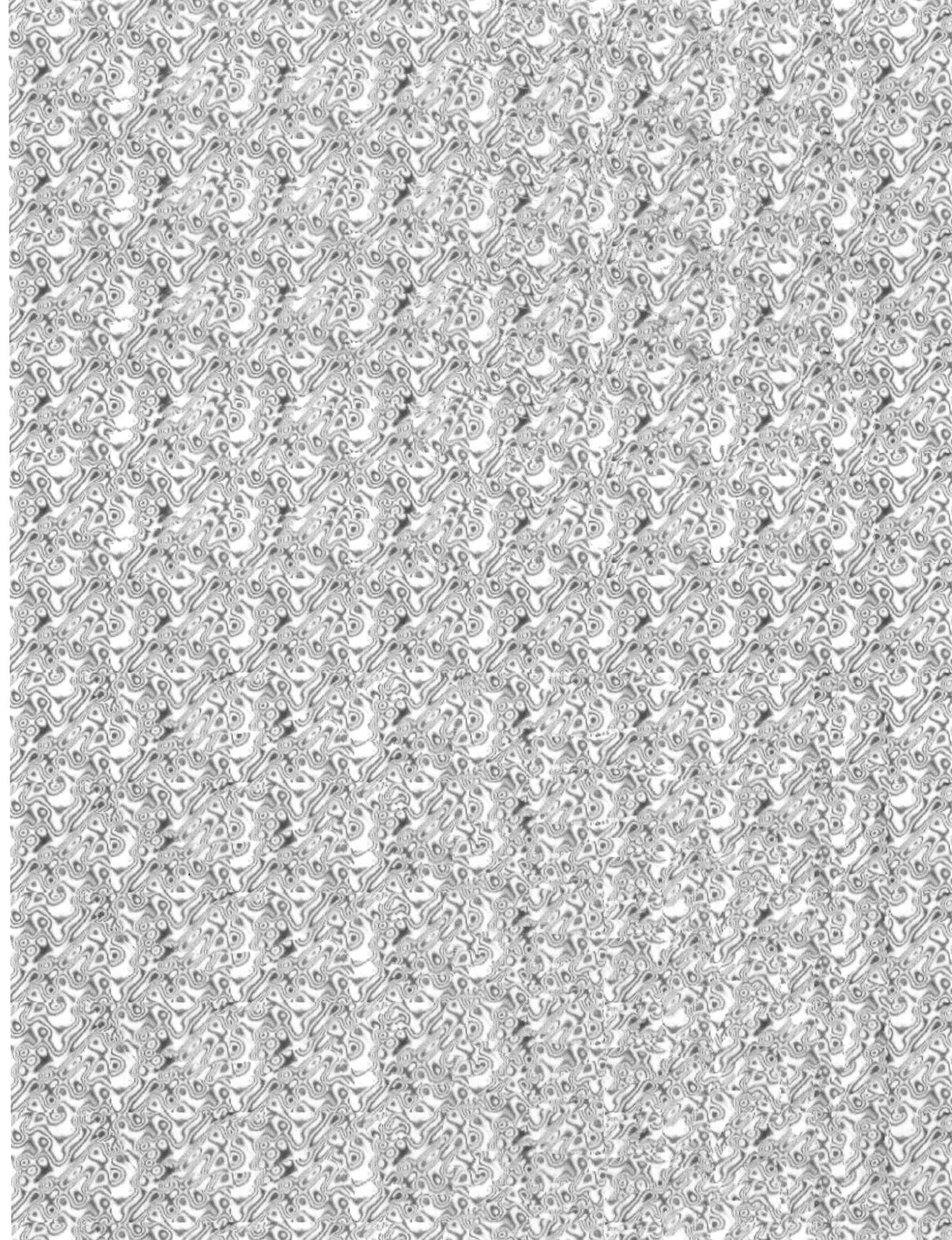

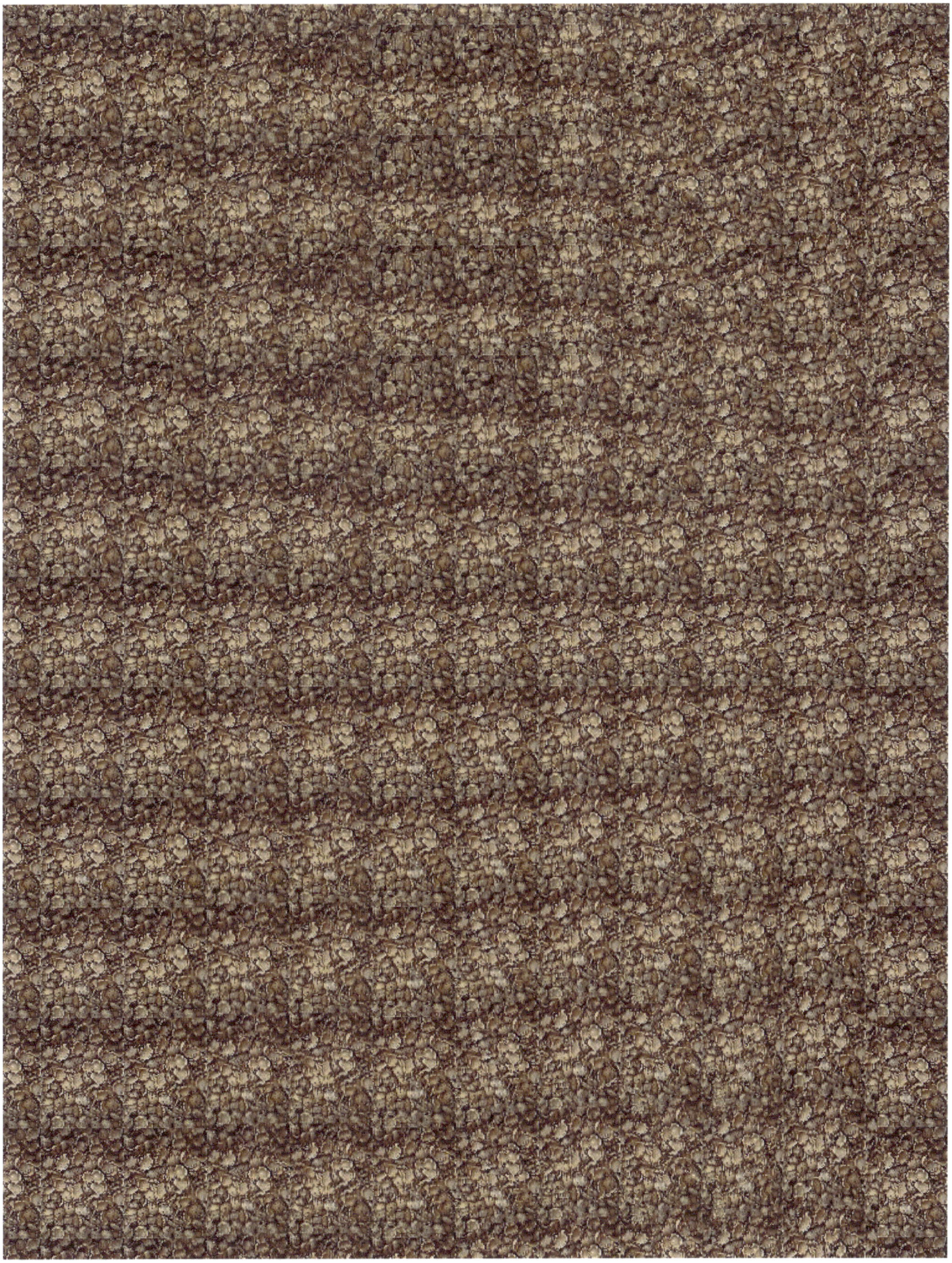

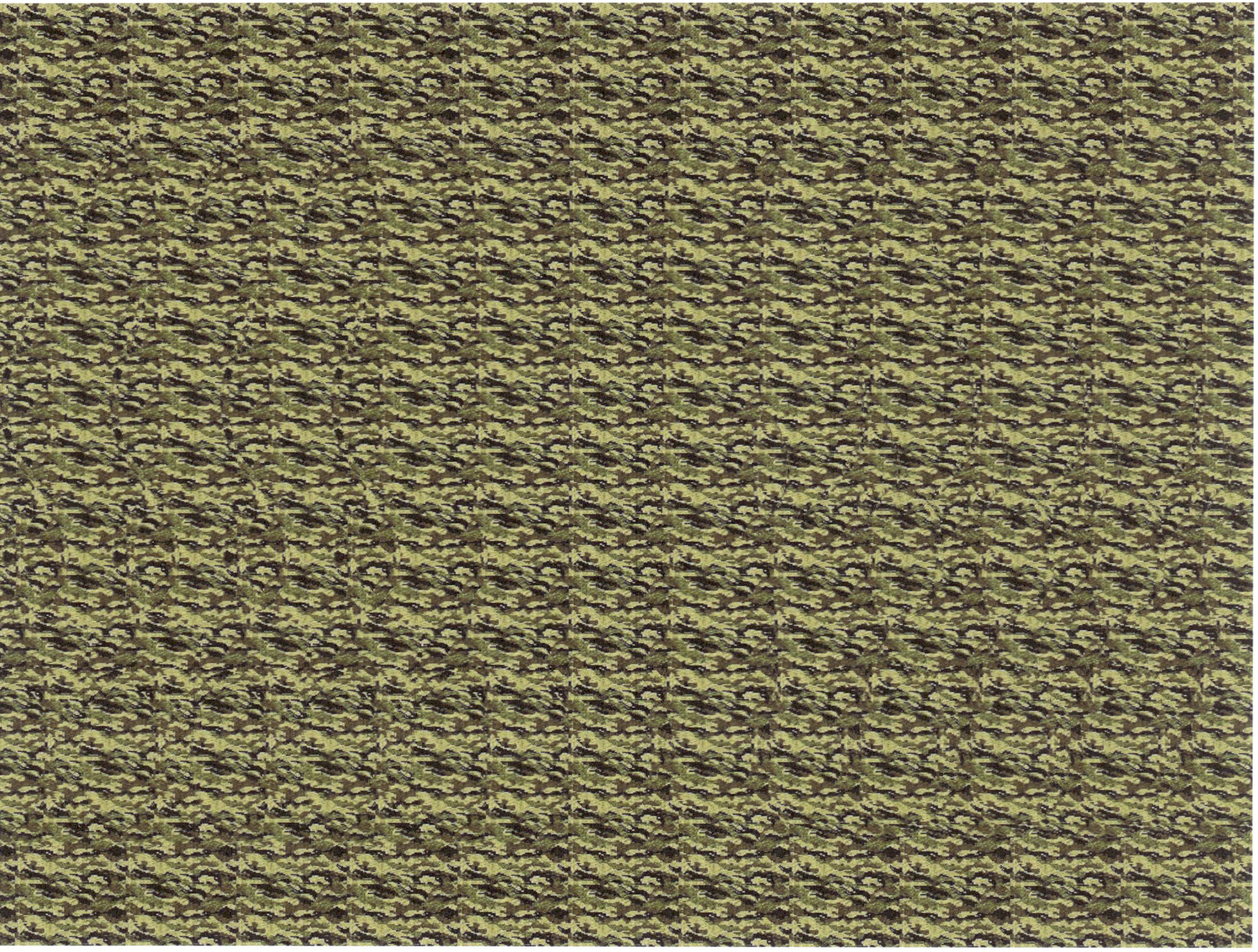

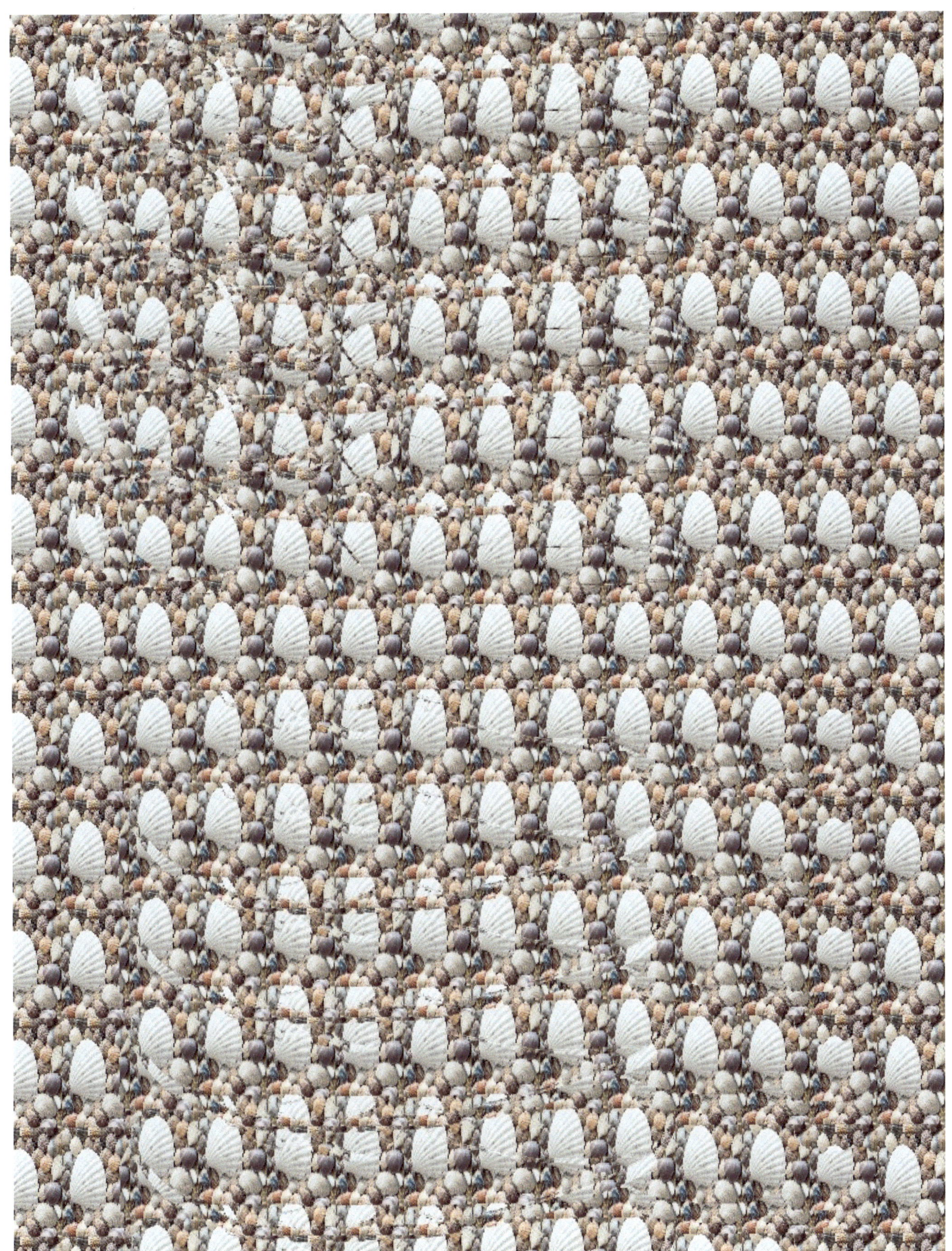

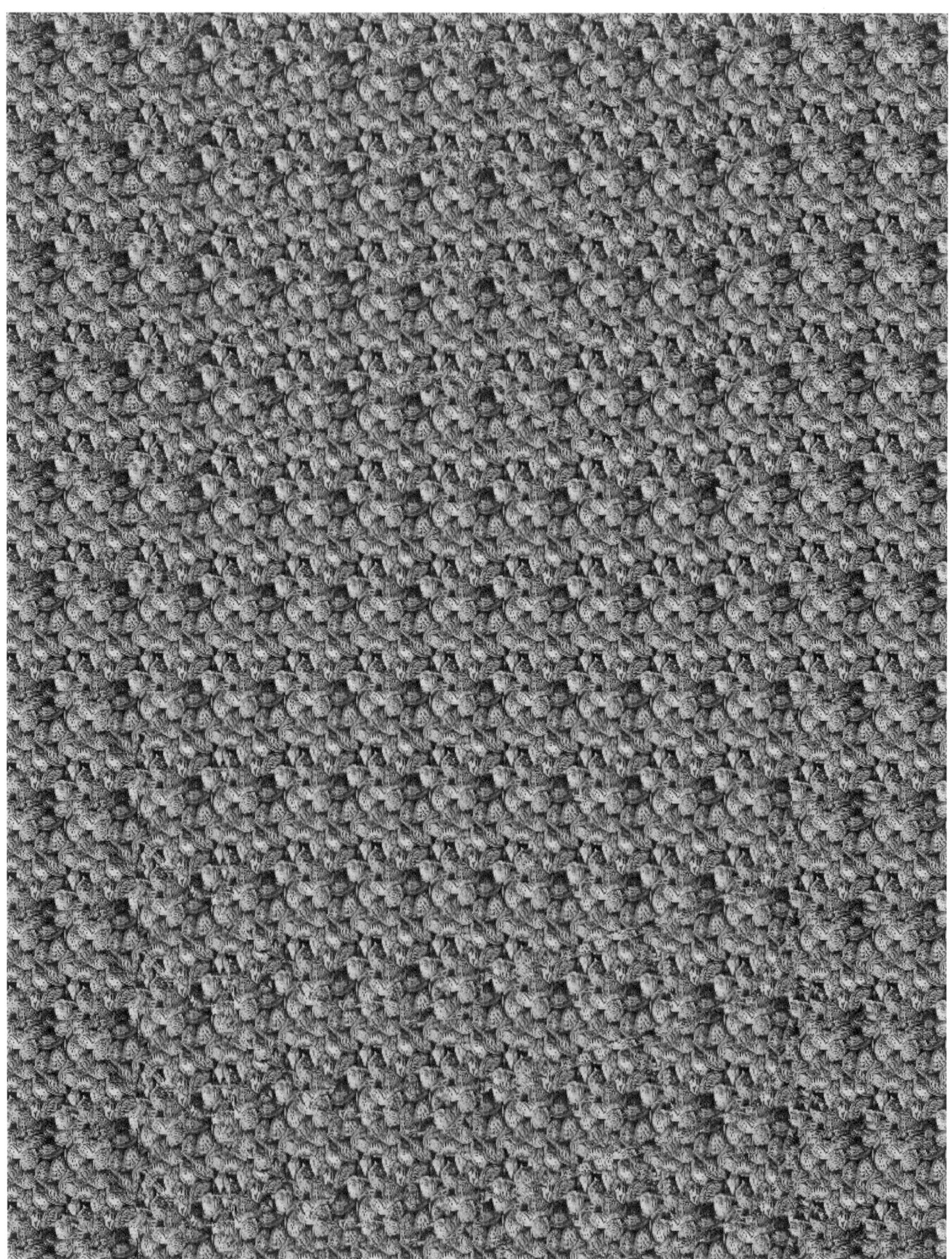

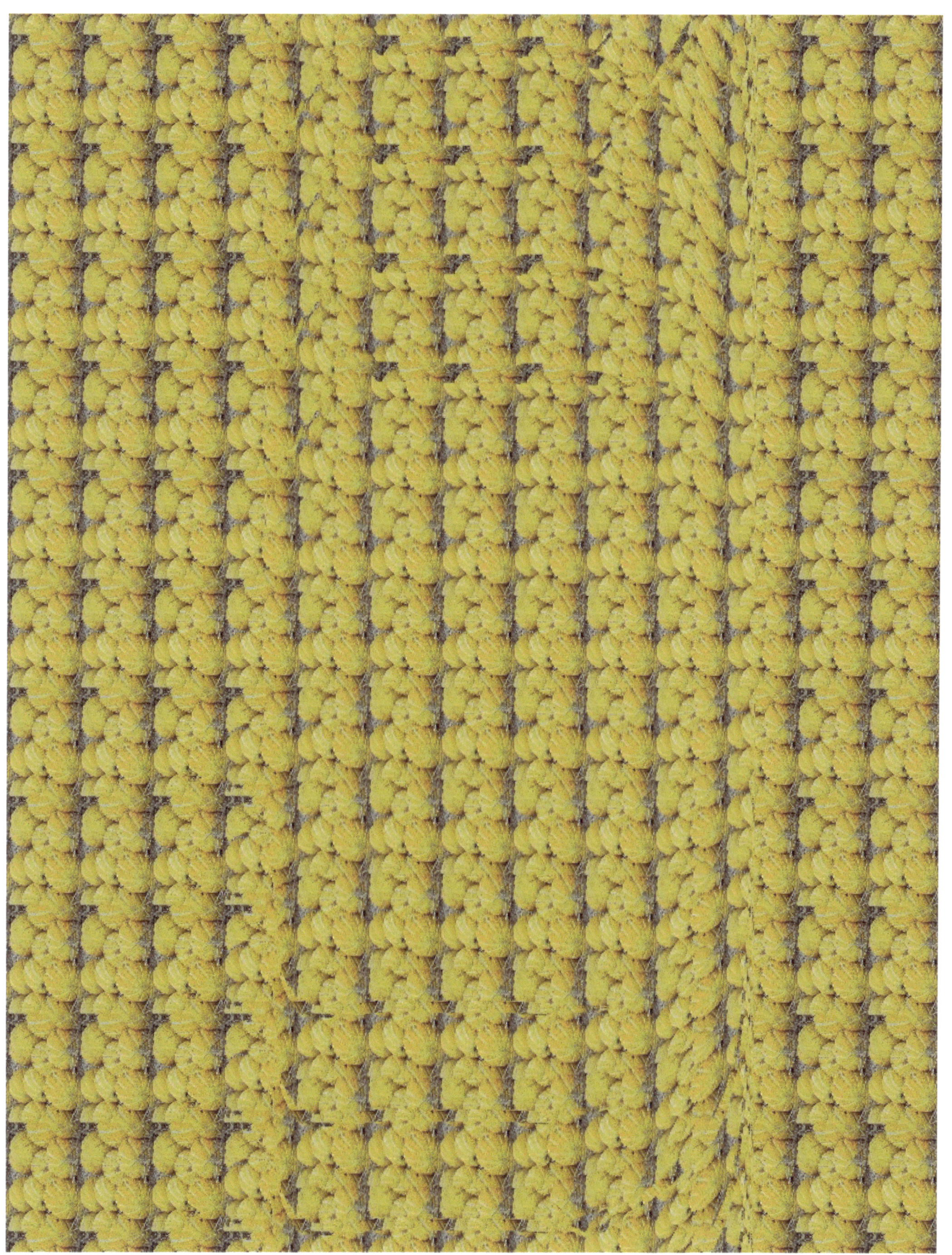

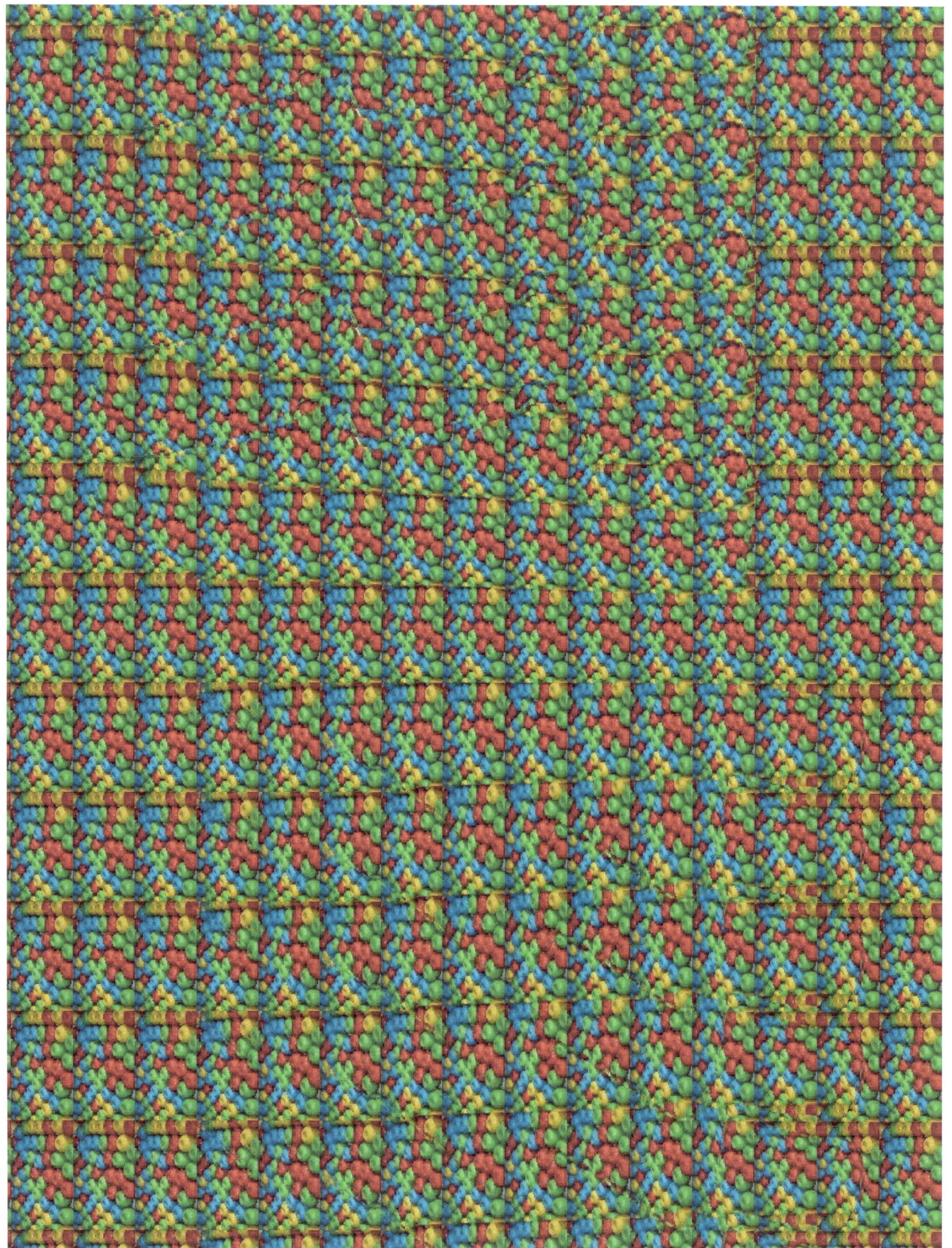

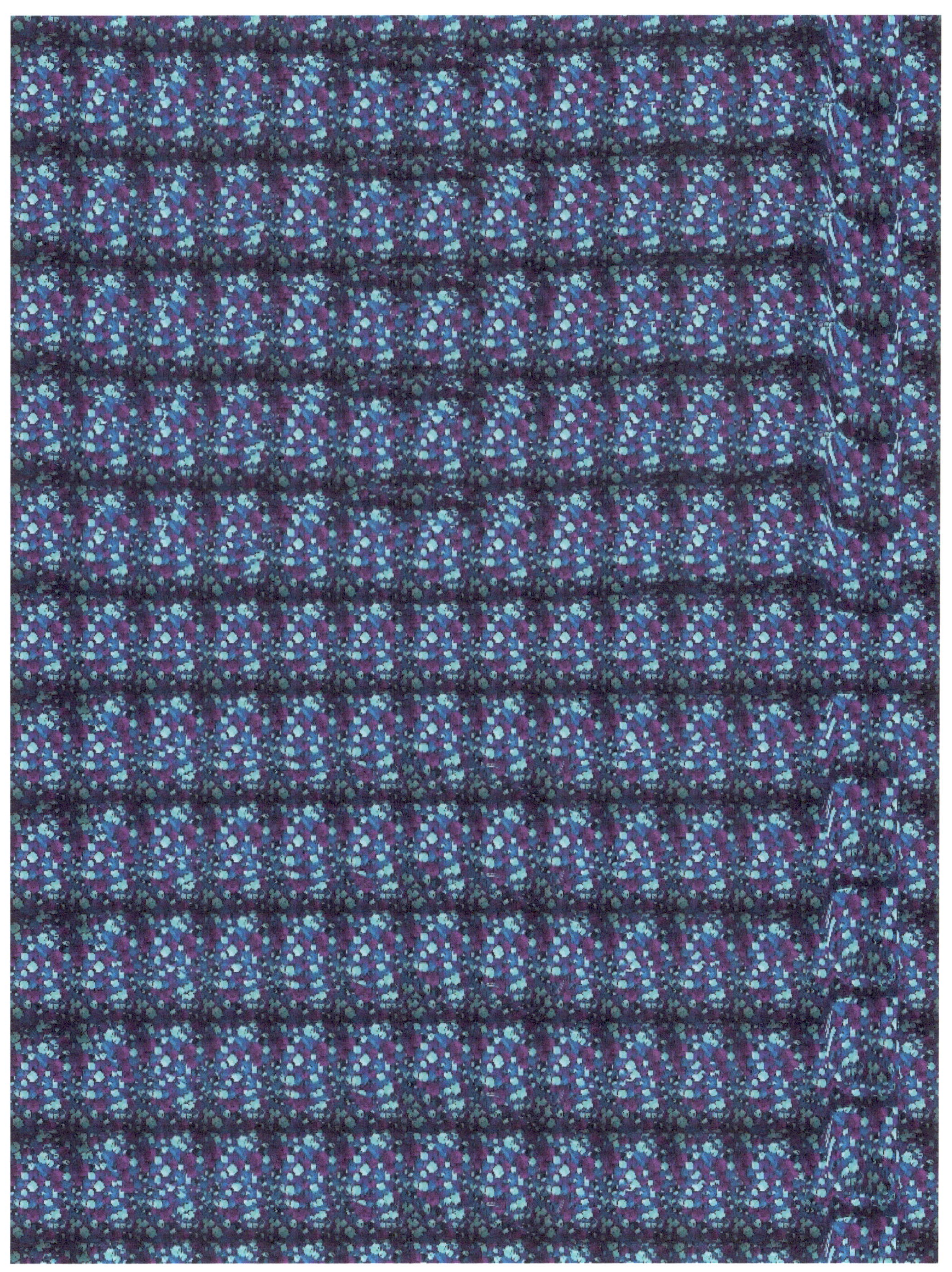

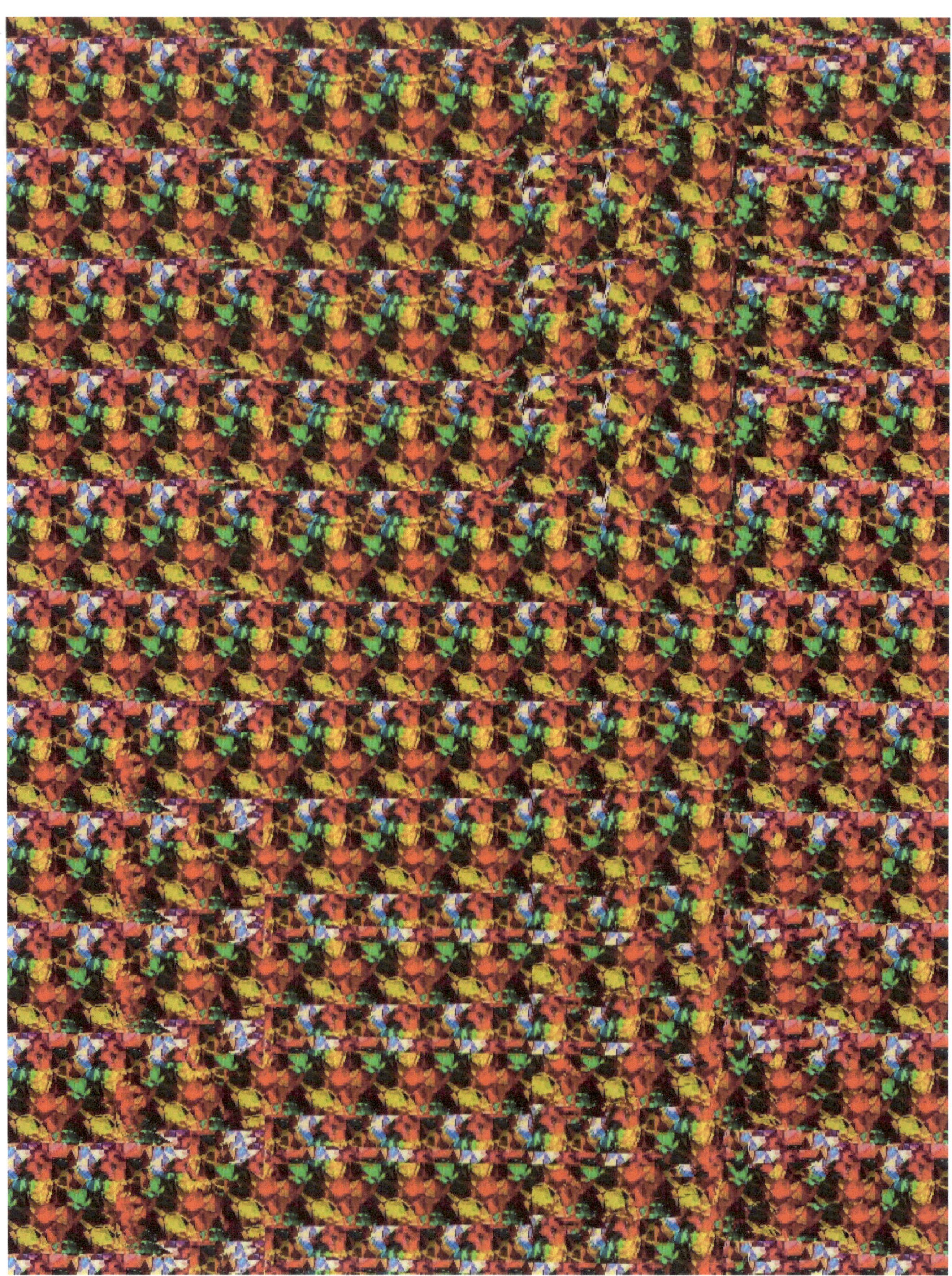

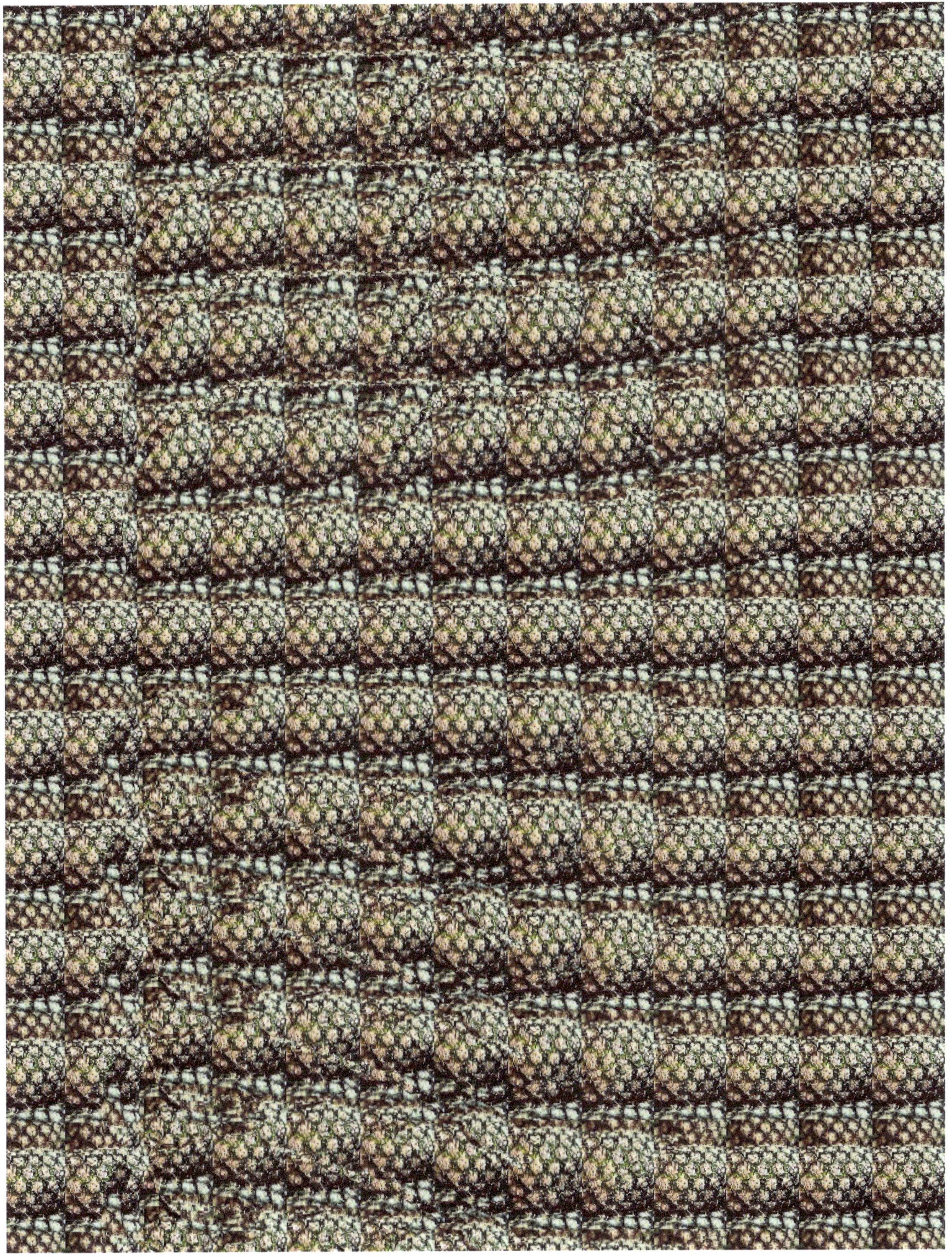

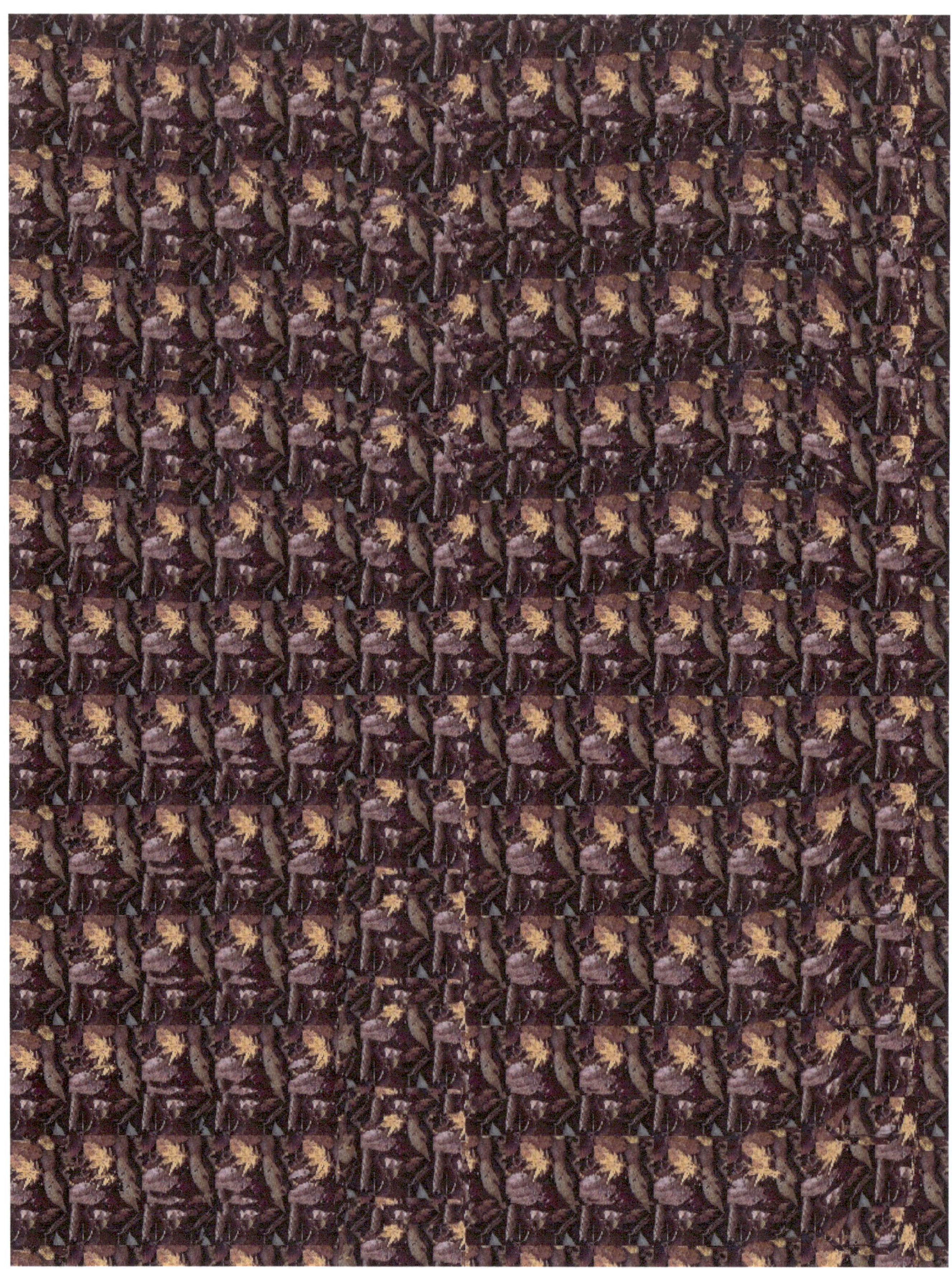

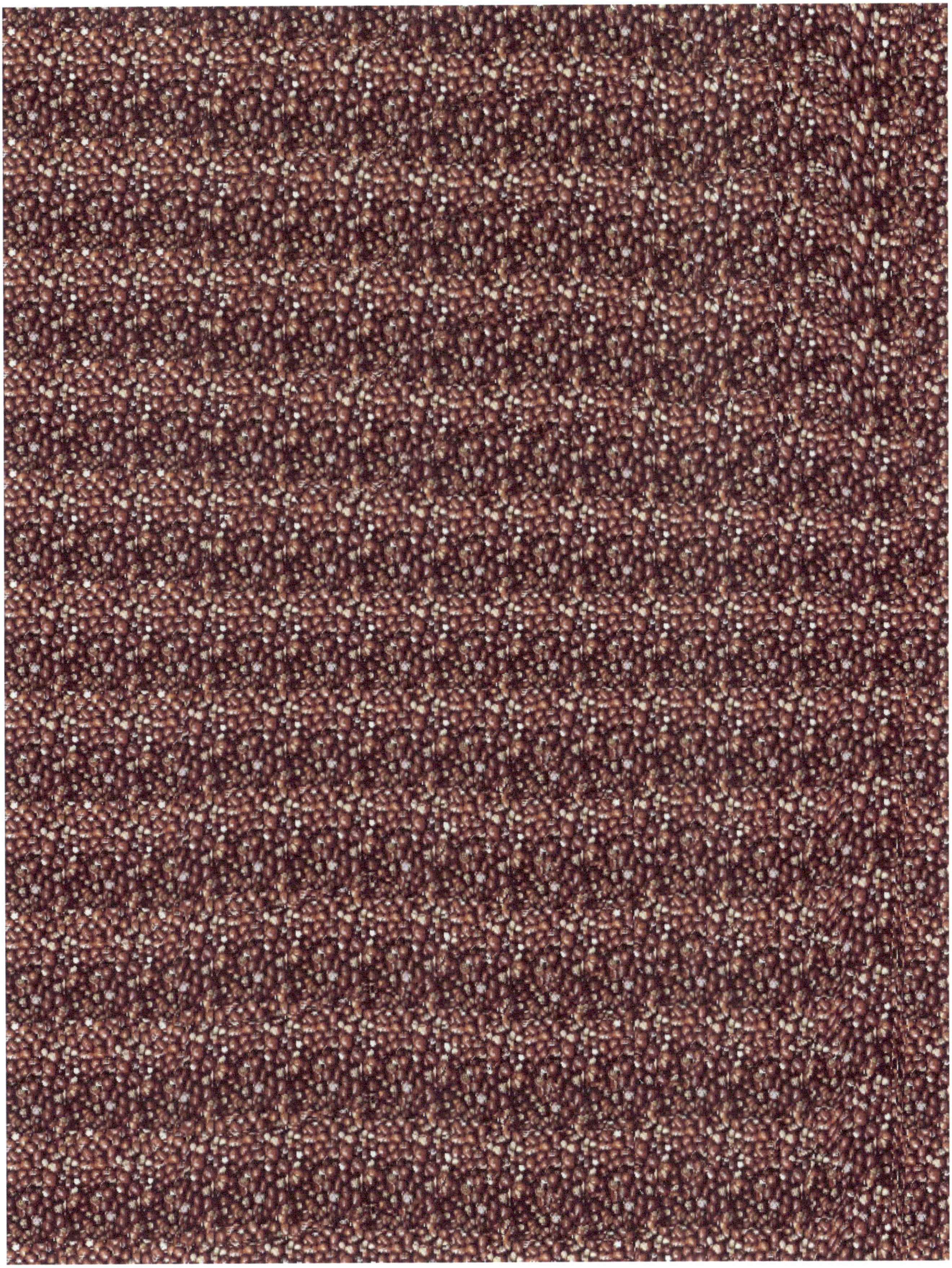

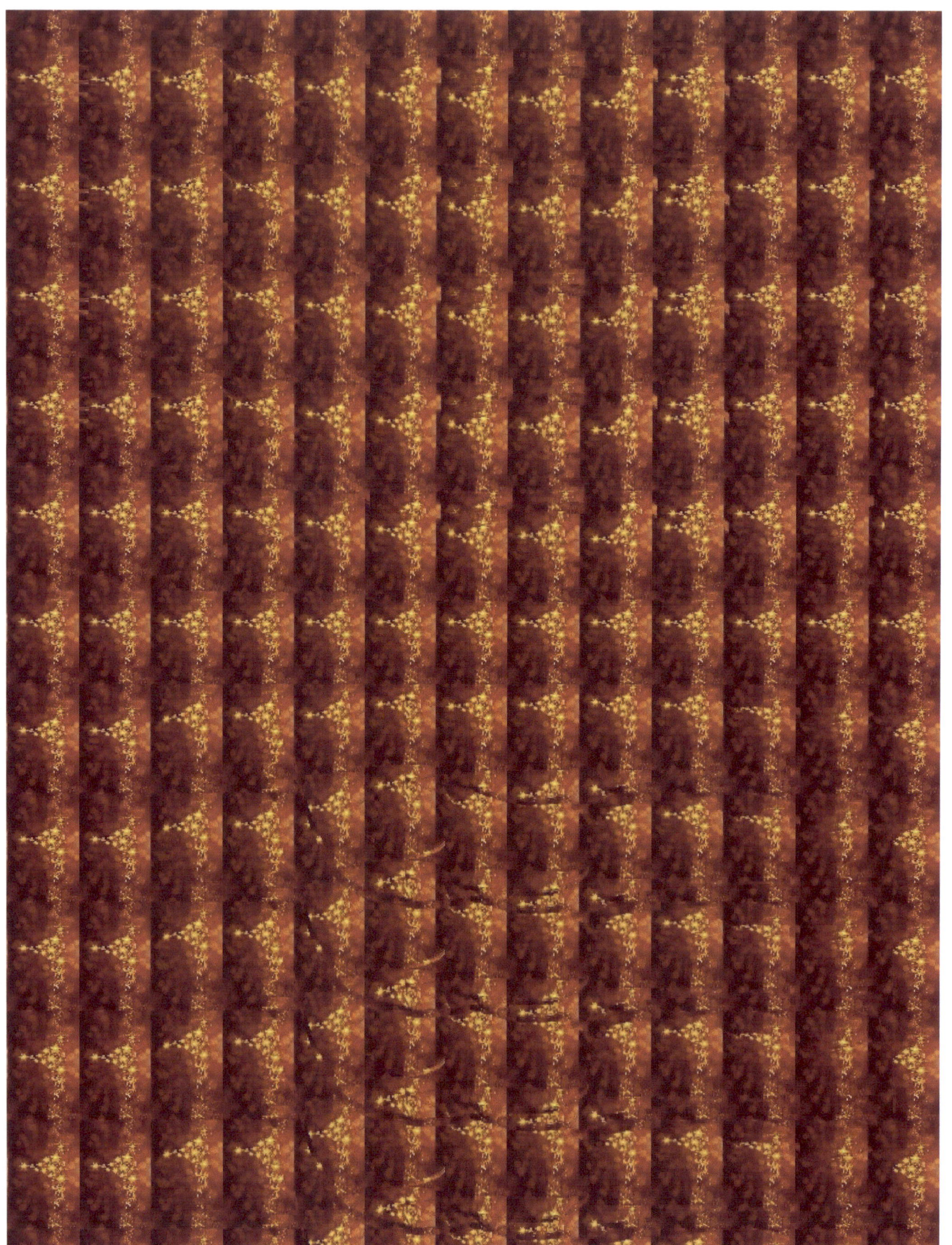

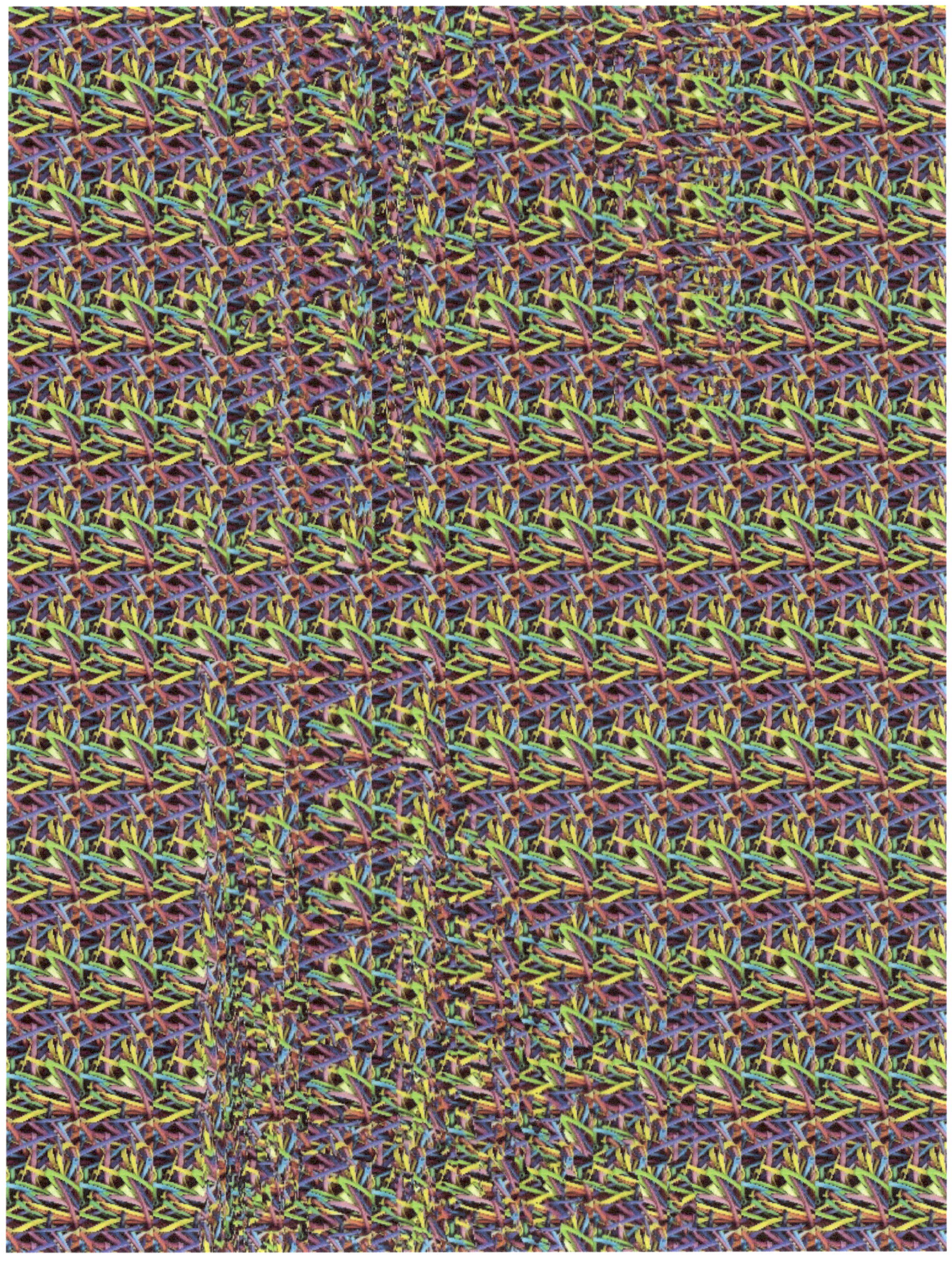

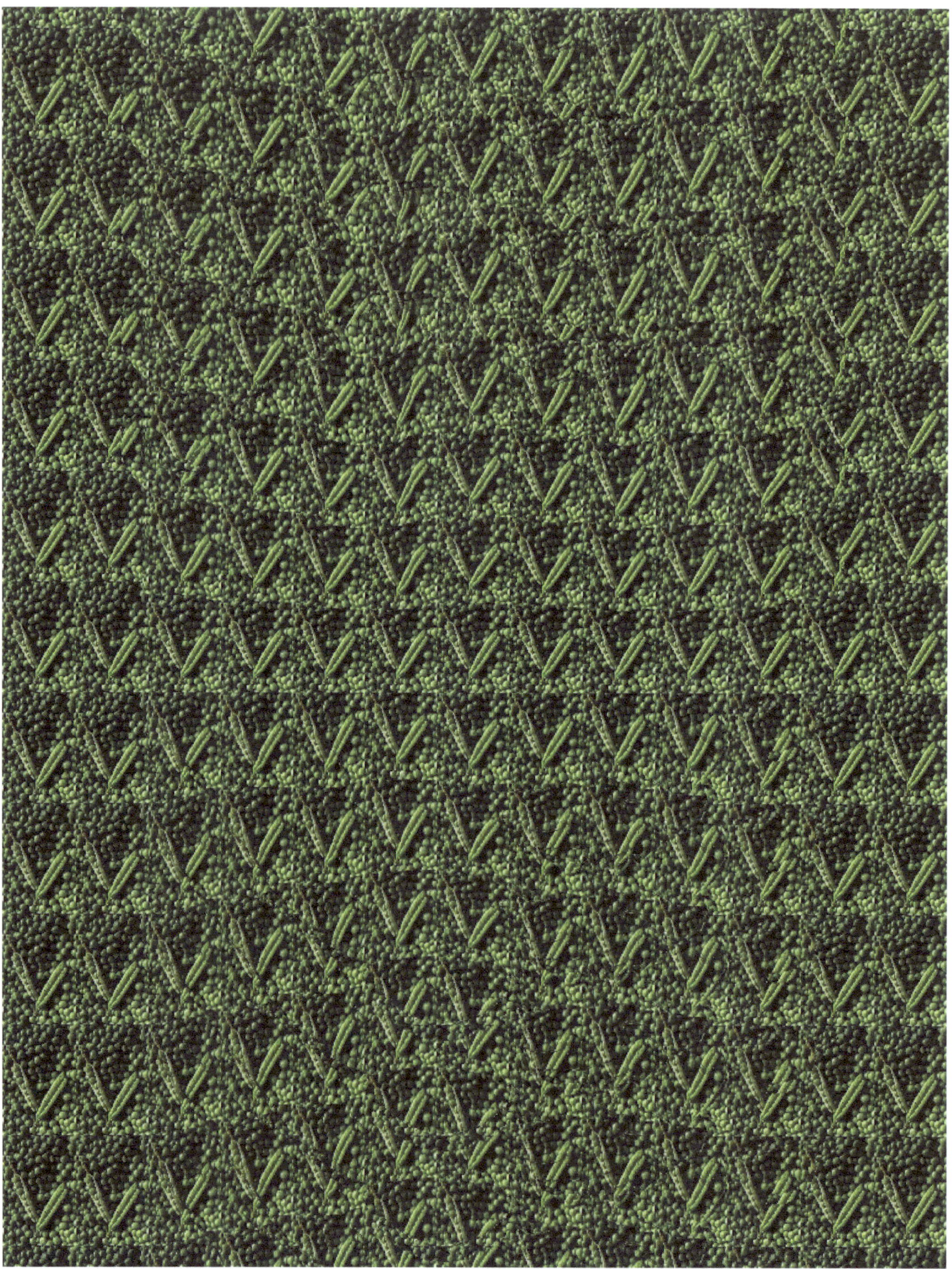

Solutions

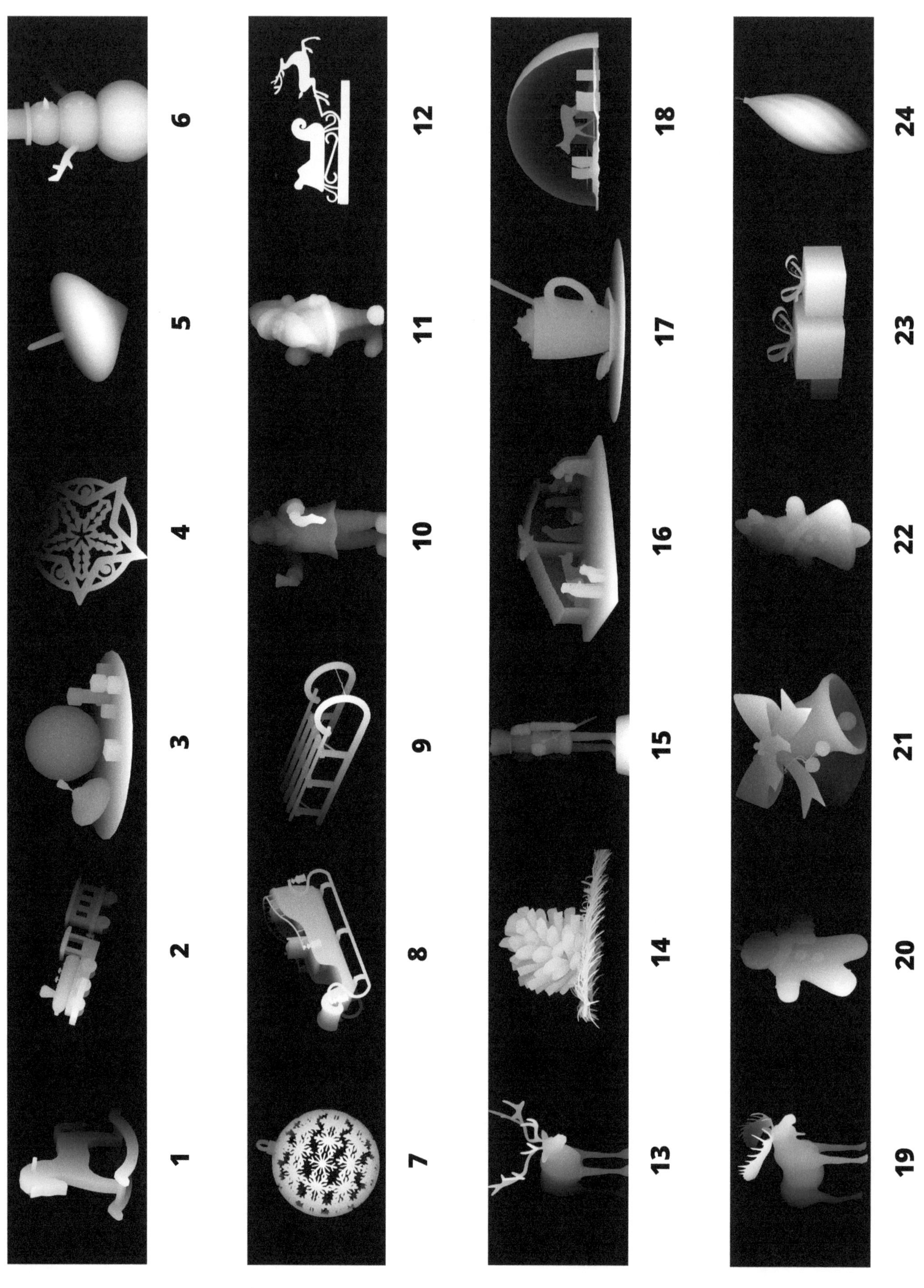

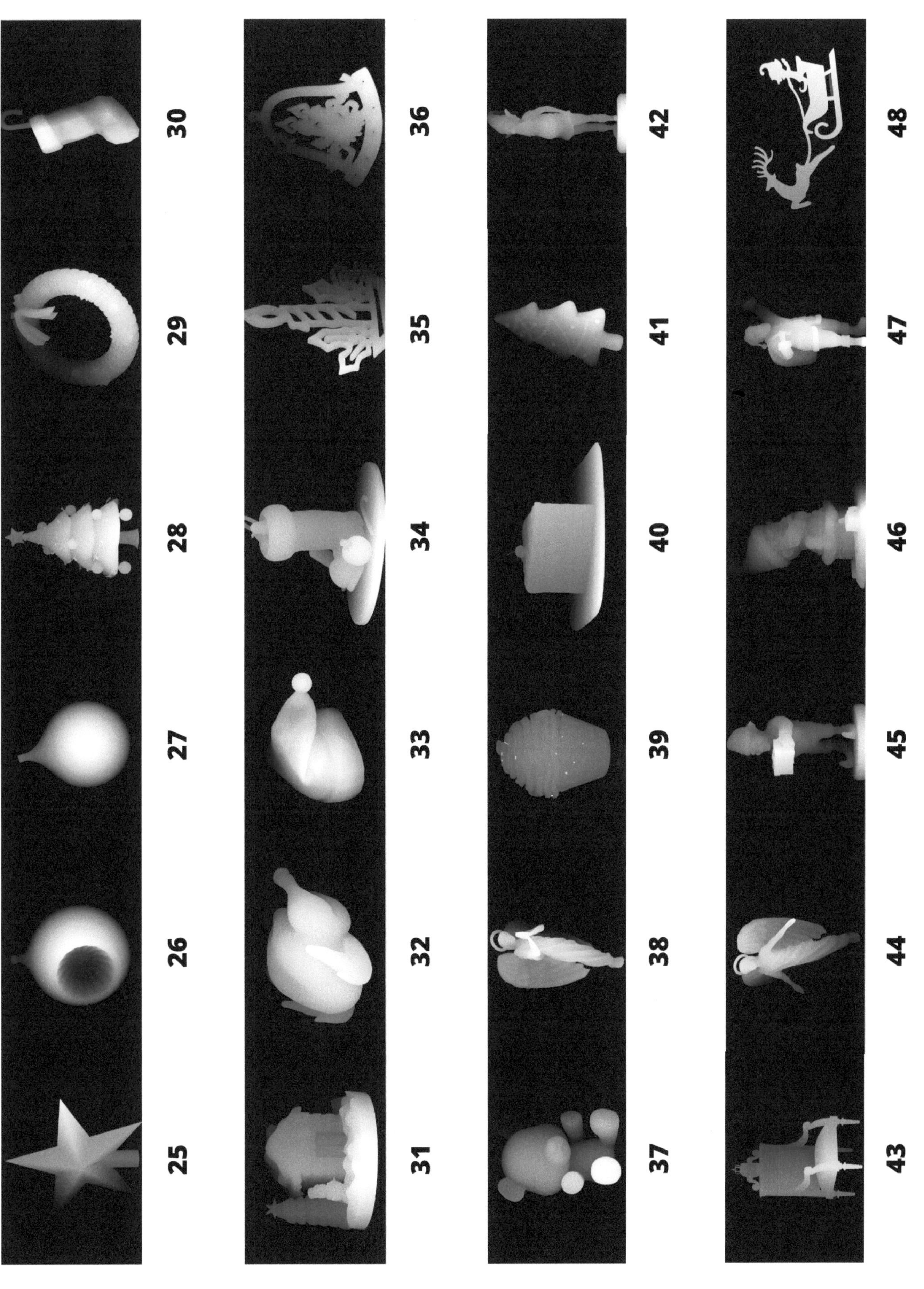

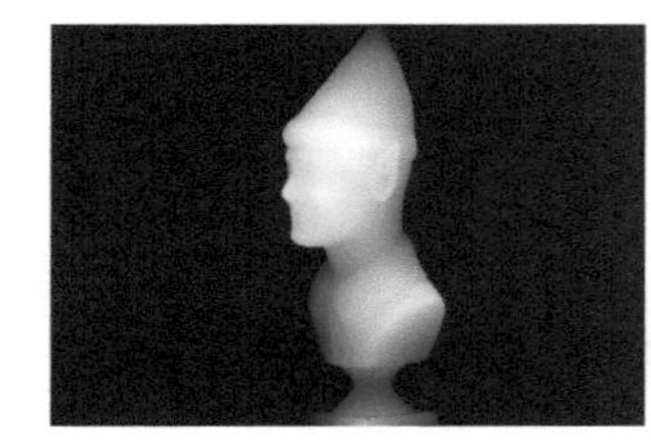

49

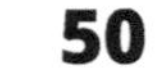

50

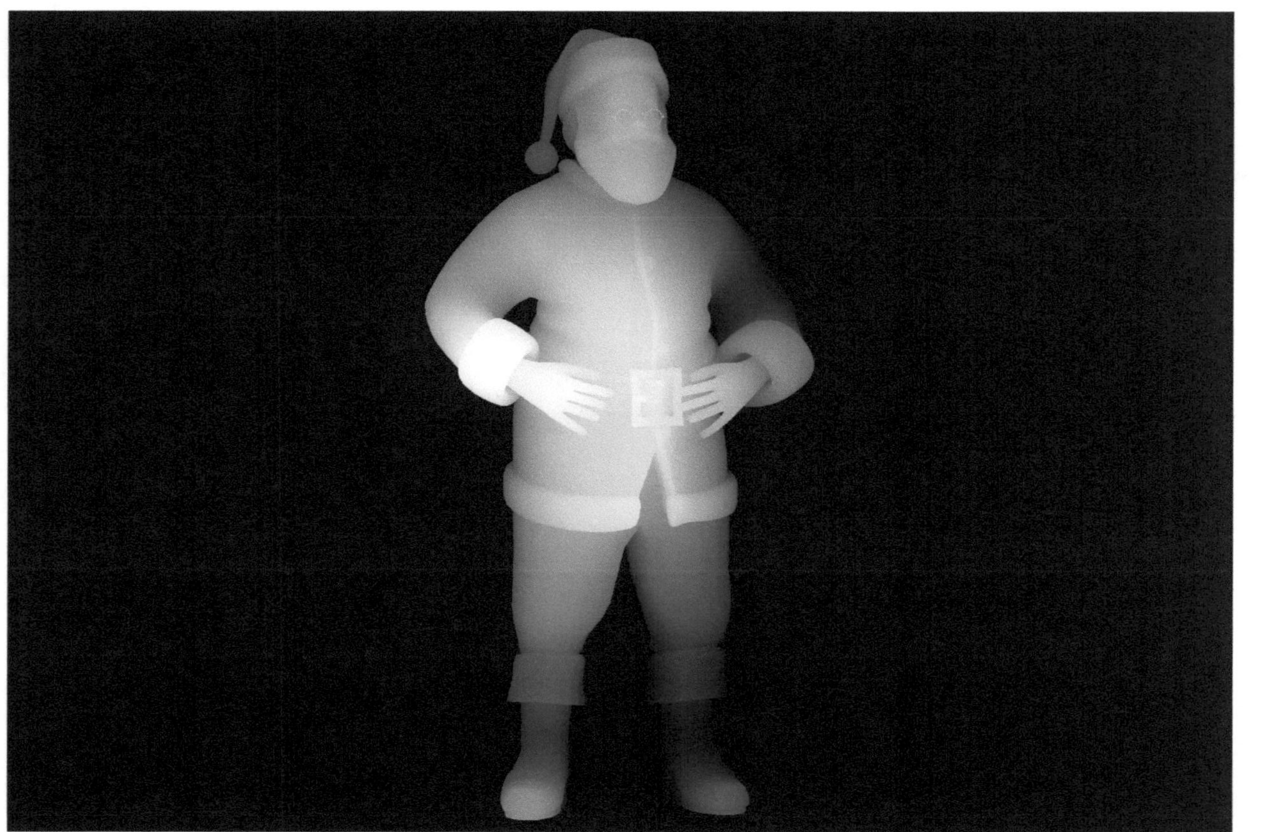

Cover image

www.ingramcontent.com/pod-product-compliance
Lightning Source LLC
Chambersburg PA
CBHW040047240726
48664CB00004B/1094